MW01029320

"Quitting alcohol is one of the most impactful decisions I've made in my adult life and James is one of the foremost experts on the topic."

— MARK MANSON,
#1 NYT bestselling author of
*The Subtle Art of Not Giving a F*ck*

"CLEAR is an essential resource for high achievers committed to living a healthier, more focused life."

— KEITH FERRAZZI,
#1 NYT bestselling author of *Never Eat Alone*

"A thought-provoking and insightful read, CLEAR offers practical advice for those seeking change."

— MAX LUGAVERE,
NYT bestselling author of *Genius Foods*

"In CLEAR, James Swanwick challenges the norms around drinking, revealing how even casual alcohol use dulls focus, drains energy, and limits success. With science-backed insights and practical strategies, this book empowers you to break free from the habit loop, unlock peak performance, and live a clearer, more vibrant life."

— NIR EYAL,
author of *Indistractable*

"James offers a compelling case for cutting out alcohol, showing how it can restore your health, strengthen immunity, and help you live at your peak."

— DR. AMY MYERS,
NYT bestselling author of *The Autoimmune Solution*

"James delivers a powerful message about alcohol in CLEAR that is both timely and necessary."

— ROBB WOLF,
NYT bestselling author of *The Paleo Solution*

"Thriving without alcohol is a super power. James Swanwick has put together an epic guide to help those who need to change their relationship with alcohol."

— JAMES SCHRAMKO,
author of *Work Less Make More*

"The tools inside CLEAR can help anybody struggling with alcohol regain their power, improve their health and transform their life. James absolutely nailed this!"

— DANIEL DIPIAZZA,
author of *Rich20Something*

"CLEAR is a must-read for anyone looking to have a better relationship with alcohol and better relationships in general."

— GINA SWIRE,
author of *PS I Love Me: 12 Steps for a Self-Love Transformation*

"CLEAR delivers a wake-up call to high achievers, showing how life without alcohol can be the ultimate competitive advantage."

— DR. MICHAEL BREUS,
author of *The Power of When*

"CLEAR offers a refreshing perspective on alcohol, with insights that are both profound and actionable."

— JOHN GRAY,
author of *Men Are from Mars, Women Are from Venus*

"Once you become alcohol-free, you'll uncover the root causes of many of the biggest challenges in your life. CLEAR is an essential guide for everyone on the journey of true personal evolution."

— JORDAN HARBINGER,
Host of *The Jordan Harbinger Show*

"The insights James reveals in CLEAR can be transformative for those who seek to change their relationship with alcohol."

— RYAN DANIEL MORAN,
author of *12 Months to $1 Million*

A NEW WAVE PRESS BOOK

ISBN (paperback): 979-8-9925418-0-9
ISBN (hardcover): 979-8-9925418-1-6
ISBN (ebook): 979-8-9925418-2-3
ISBN (audiobook): 979-8-9925418-3-0

Printed in The United States of America

*Clear: The Only Neuroscience-Based Method for High Achievers
to Quit Drinking Without Willpower, Rehab or AA*

© 2025 James Swanwick
All Rights Reserved

New Wave Press values and upholds copyright, recognizing it as a
driving force behind creativity, diverse perspectives, and the free exchange of ideas. By purchasing an authorized edition of this book and
respecting copyright laws—refraining from reproducing, scanning, or
distributing any portion without permission—you are directly supporting authors and enabling New Wave Press to continue bringing
impactful books to readers everywhere. Thank you for being part of
this creative ecosystem.

Although every effort has been made to ensure that the personal and
professional advice present within this book is useful and appropriate, the author and publisher do not assume and hereby disclaim any
liability to any person, business, or organization choosing to employ
the guidance offered in this book.

This is a work of nonfiction. All people, locations, events, and situations are portrayed to the best of the author's memory.

No part of this book may be reproduced, stored in a retrieval system,
or transmitted by any means without the written permission of the
author and publisher.

New Wave Press
New York • Los Angeles
newwavepress.co

clear

THE ONLY NEUROSCIENCE-BASED METHOD
FOR HIGH ACHIEVERS TO QUIT DRINKING
WITHOUT WILLPOWER, REHAB OR AA

JAMES SWANWICK

WITH DANIEL DIPIAZZA

*Dedicated to my mother and father,
Jill and Ron Swanwick;*

my beautiful partner, Laura;

*and all those with the courage to choose
an alcohol-free lifestyle.*

TABLE OF CONTENTS

Introduction..xii

PART I
Rewriting Your Story About Alcohol....................1

CHAPTER 1: Why We Drink...................................3

CHAPTER 2: How to Refocus Your
           Mindset Around Alcohol 39

PART II:
The Case for Going Alcohol-Free...................... 67

CHAPTER 3: Healing the Effects of
           Alcohol on Your Brain and Body.............. 69

CHAPTER 4: Upgrade Your Epigenetics 93

CHAPTER 5: How Eliminating Alcohol
           Grows Your Business and Your Wealth 109

CHAPTER 6: Deepen Your Connections
           without Alcohol............................ 125

PART III:

Beginning Your Alcohol-Free Lifestyle 159

CHAPTER 7: Cultivating Sustainable Joy 161

CHAPTER 8: Your Step-by-Step Action
Plan to Becoming Alcohol-Free.............. 177

CHAPTER 9: Embracing the Uncomfortable
Clarity of Your New Reality................. 195

Acknowledgments 215

About the Authors 219

Appendix A: Twenty-Two Delicious
Alcohol-Free Drink Recipes 223

Appendix B: AFL Research Study........................ 231

Notes 237

Index.. 243

INTRODUCTION

I F YOU'RE READING THIS BOOK, you may be at a crossroads in your life. Something needs to change with your relationship to alcohol and you've known it for a long time. If you've been waiting for a sign, this is it.

If your personal or professional relationships are suffering because of your drinking and it's been this way for a decade or more, there's a real danger you could lose everything. You could lose your marriage. You could lose your business or career. You could lose your relationship with your children or grandchildren. You could lose your health. You could lose your life. You may have lost some of these already.

Alcohol can cause you to disconnect from your friends and loved ones. It can cause you to neglect yourself for years. It's one of the biggest reasons clients in our *Project* 90 quit drinking program say they don't feel as present with their kids or partner as they'd like.

The good news is, you can take your power back from alcohol for good. In fact, you've already taken the first step by reading this book. The next step is to implement what you learn in the coming chapters. You can choose to be alcohol-free, starting today, even if you've tried and failed in the past. Especially if you've tried and failed already.

How can I be so certain? The difference is that this time around you'll have access to the systems and tools we teach at Alcohol-Free Lifestyle (AFL), which have been demonstrated to reduce alcohol consumption by 98 percent over ninety days according to a study conducted at the University of Washington in 2023. That study is reproduced in the appendix at the back of this book for your reference. We know what works.

Recently, our team interviewed a successful attorney who said she felt trapped and exhausted from her alcohol habit of over ten years. She shared with us that she didn't feel present with her two kids or focused with her clients. She wanted to set a better example for her family. She wanted to feel healthier. She knew that needed to change.

We spoke with a surgeon who has been drinking heavily for thirteen years. He said he drinks a bottle of red wine every night, sometimes more. He drinks to deal with stress. He thinks about drinking when he's not drinking. He thinks about how he can hide alcohol with him when he goes out places where drinking isn't allowed. He doesn't feel in control. He wants to quit drinking, but he's scared of what life will look like without alcohol.

We also heard from a vice president at a technology firm who was regularly drinking seven to eight beers a night during the week and sometimes more on the weekends. He told us that he felt that he was letting his wife down and that he was disappointed with himself. He wanted to quit drinking, but didn't know how else he was going to deal with all the stress from work.

These are the types of people who come into the AFL community and are successful with the systems you're about to learn. Just like you, they're high performers, but they're not perfect. Just like you, alcohol is causing them and their families massive pain. Just like you, they've probably tried to change their alcohol habits before and have always gone back to it. Just like you, they've reached a breaking point.

I challenge you to make a mental note of the time and day you're reading this book. Now, mark it in your mind as the moment you finally decided to transform your life.

If you're committed to that change, what you read in this book will help you break free of the grip of alcohol for good—as it has for over 3,000 successful clients in the Alcohol-Free Lifestyle community.

We don't use traditional 12-step methodology in our programs. We don't simply use motivation or inspiration. We don't focus on seasonal challenges like "Sober October" or "Dry January." We definitely don't "white knuckle" it. Our approach is based on science and data of what works in the real world. We support lifelong change with the only neuroscience-based method for high achievers to quit drinking. What you'll learn in this book will literally rewire your brain, if you let it.

You have two options from here: you can continue down the road you're on, knowing where it leads. Or you can choose the alcohol-free road. The road without alcohol is certainly the one less traveled in today's culture. It can be challenging, lonely and scary at times. But once you take it, you're on the path to freedom, happiness, peace of mind, and longevity.

Keep reading and take another step in that direction.

HOW TO TELL IF YOU HAVE ALCOHOL USE DISORDER (AUD)

Let's get one thing clear: you're not an "alcoholic." To many, this word is an outdated label that not only feels derogatory and inherently judgmental—it also fails to account for the fact that alcohol use exists on a spectrum and your relationship with it can change over time. Addictions are not black and white or static.

The term being used by modern medicine and in the Alcohol-Free Lifestyle community to describe an addictive pattern with alcohol is *alcohol use disorder* (AUD). This classification allows for the fact that there's a broad spectrum in the severity of misuse of alcohol. It also recognizes that having AUD is not a moral failing or character flaw. Alcohol use disorder is a negative habit loop you've created with alcohol that is triggered by stress and other emotions. It's a disorder that anybody can develop over time without even realizing it's happening. Research shows that some people are up to 50 percent more likely to develop AUD than others based on family history.[1]

According to the Centers for Disease Control and Prevention (CDC), the average alcohol consumption per week among American adults varies by gender. Men, on average, consume about two drinks per day, while women typically consume one drink per day on average.[2] That's an average of about 700 drinks per year from men and 350 per year for women — 7,000 and 3,500 drinks per decade, respectively. Terrifyingly, these figures represent thresholds for what has been considered "normal" drinking according to U.S. health standards. Until now.

In January 2025, the U.S. surgeon general, Dr. Vivek Murthy, declared alcohol was a leading preventable cause of cancer. He called for alcoholic beverages to carry a warning label, as packs of cigarettes do. It was the latest in a fierce debate about the risks and so-called benefits of moderate drinking.

Do you regularly have more than one to two drinks per day? If so, you may have some level of alcohol use disorder. AFL coach Victoria English shared something about her "awakening" around alcohol that really struck me:

> *When I began to struggle with my drinking in my thirties, I would go online and look at the "Are you an alcoholic?" quiz. And in the beginning, I only checked a couple of those boxes. It never occurred to me that I had permission to question my relationship with alcohol at that point.*
>
> *Six months later, I go back to that quiz, and I check another box. A year later, I was checking more boxes, and that's when I said "Well, I guess it's bad enough." I think that's a really important message to destigmatize this... frame it as an opportunity for growth... most people don't even know they have the permission to question until they're checking a lot of those boxes.*

This hit me hard because, like Victoria, I didn't have a singular "rock bottom" moment. My transformation came from finally giving myself permission to examine my relationship with alcohol and make a new decision, whereas before, I hadn't even realized I had a choice.

Let's start by getting crystal clear on where you stand with alcohol.

KEY INDICATORS OF ALCOHOL USE DISORDER

You may have asked yourself before, "Am I an alcoholic?" and decided that since you didn't fit the negative stereotype, you were in the clear. However, progression from experimentation, to habit, to dependence, to addiction is slow and can be hard to recognize within yourself if you don't know what to look for. Alcohol use disorder can develop over time and live in the background of our lives, wreaking havoc for decades if left unchecked. It's good to have an objective way of looking at your own habits.

Here are the key indicators of AUD according to the DSM-V[3], which classifies psychological diseases and conditions. The severity of AUD is determined based on the presence of these symptoms. The more of these you have, the higher the severity.

Read through them and make an honest assessment about how many apply to you.

In the past year, have you:

1. Had times when you ended up drinking more, or longer, than you intended?
2. More than once wanted to cut down or stop drinking, or tried to but couldn't?
3. Spent a lot of time drinking? Or being sick or getting over other aftereffects?
4. Wanted a drink so badly you couldn't think of anything else?

5. Found that drinking—or being sick from drinking—often interfered with taking care of your home or family? Or caused job troubles? Or school problems?
6. Continued to drink even though it was causing trouble with your family or friends?
7. Given up or cut back on activities that were important or interesting or gave you pleasure, in order to drink?
8. More than once gotten into situations while or after drinking that increased your chances of getting hurt (such as driving, swimming, using machinery, walking in a dangerous area, or having unsafe sex)?
9. Continued to drink even though it was making you feel depressed or anxious or adding to another health problem? Or after having a memory blackout?
10. Had to drink much more than you once did to get the effect you want? Or found that your usual number of drinks had much less effect than before?
11. Found that, when the effects of alcohol were wearing off, you had withdrawal symptoms, such as trouble sleeping, shakiness, restlessness, nausea, sweating, a racing heart, or a seizure? Or sensed things that were not there?

Now, check in with yourself:

» How many of the above applied to you?
» Has this list been growing or shrinking in the last year?

According to the DSM, having two to three symptoms from the above list indicates mild alcohol use disorder. Experiencing four to five symptoms indicates moderate AUD. Anything above five is severe. Many clients in the Alcohol-Free Lifestyle community are in the third category, battling severe alcohol use disorder in addition to having responsibilities at home and a demanding professional life. If that's you, you're in the right place.

QUESTIONING YOUR BELIEFS ABOUT ALCOHOL

Cultural conditioning has led us to believe that alcohol is important and that moderate or even severe drinking is a normal part of our lifestyle, never questioning how it might make us feel. But is it really natural? Or are our socially acceptable drinking habits slowly and methodically sapping our physical, mental, financial, and spiritual potential? Is alcohol really supporting our social lives, our careers, and our

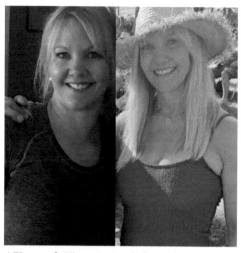

AFL coach Victoria English made a mental, physical and spiritual transformation when she finally gave herself permission to question her relationship with alcohol.

happiness? Or is it merely an attractively packaged poison that's gradually draining our inner and outer resources?

According to Nielsen data, nearly half of Americans are actively attempting to cut back on drinking. Nonalcoholic bars are opening up in hip corners of New York, London, and Los Angeles. Sales of nonalcoholic beer, wine, and cocktails have skyrocketed, with dozens of new brands popping up to meet the increased consumer demand. The alcohol-alternative beverage market has exploded over the last decade and is now expected to exceed $29 billion by 2026. Even Budweiser has jumped on the bandwagon, debuting an alcohol-free beer, Budweiser Zero, in July 2020.

Some of the world's most successful people have made the conscious choice to embrace the alcohol-free lifestyle, including billionaires like Warren Buffett, Michael Dell, and Larry Ellison; business leaders like Ariana Huffington and Tom's Shoes founder Blake Mycoskie; thought leaders like Tony Robbins and Brené Brown (who calls living alcohol-free her "superpower"); and

Hollywood stars like Bradley Cooper, Natalie Portman, Pharrell Williams, and Jennifer Lopez.

The simple truth is that alcohol is toxic to our system, and we take a little hit with every drink we consume. By the time we're in our forties, if not earlier, our bodies and minds begin to reflect the cumulative impact. I often say that it's difficult to fully appreciate how damaging alcohol is because it's death by a thousand cuts. It's an invisible, gradual deterioration—an energy faucet slowly leaking until suddenly you're tired all the time, gaining unwanted weight, losing focus and motivation, and leaving your potential on the table. There's a snowball effect that, over the years, adds up to huge losses in performance, success, business revenue, personal income, happiness, and fulfillment.

For professional high performers, these losses can be especially detrimental and discouraging. If you run your own business, drinking alcohol might translate into not closing a deal because you're too foggy and lethargic. On a more subtle level, those extra five to ten pounds might leave you feeling just a little less confident. You lose your edge. Customers and potential clients go elsewhere because you weren't at the top of your game.

More importantly, these effects often trickle down into your family and personal life. You may feel less willing to try new things or spend time with loved ones unless alcohol is involved. You may find yourself more worried about your health than normal because of your drinking habit. You may find yourself struggling to do anything but sit on the couch and drink when you're not at work and not liking the person you see in the mirror.

It's time to change that, starting now.

MY ALCOHOL-FREE BREAKTHROUGH

My defining moment came on March 11, 2010. I was thirty-four. I awoke in my Austin, Texas, hotel room with a mild hangover after a night of two gin and tonics at a South by Southwest festival party. I looked in the mirror, noticed the bags under my eyes and the fat rolls hanging over my briefs, and tasted my dry mouth. It wasn't rock bottom, but in that moment, I felt the mediocrity of my life. I was stuck in a drift, heading in the direction of average. I was leaving my potential on the table.

I walked next door to IHOP for a "hangover breakfast." The sight of those scrambled eggs and bacon on the colorful, laminated menu, and people around me scarfing down piles of syrupy pancakes, made my hangover feel all the worse. I looked out the window and had one of those unremarkable but life-changing moments of clarity: this wasn't how I wanted to be living my life. I'd had enough of feeling average. Of being average. Right then and there, I resolved to give up alcohol for thirty days. It was a personal challenge to test my self-discipline and see if I could make it through.

When I started that thirty-day challenge, I had no idea it would become a new lifestyle.

The first week felt challenging at times but not nearly as much as I'd feared. I noticed I was a little more irritable. I tossed and turned slightly more during the night. But I certainly didn't experience dramatic withdrawal symptoms of migraines or night sweats that I'd been culturally conditioned to fear.

The more challenging part of the first week was actually the social element. It initially felt awkward turning up at a bar or restaurant and ordering a soda water because I feared interrogation from friends. I was surprised that some people didn't even notice and others didn't seem to care. Those who did notice jokingly gave me a hard time. I got a lot of quips like, "You're so un-Australian." I just smiled and laughed with them. By week two, I started feeling better, sleeping more deeply and noticing that I had more mental clarity.

After the first thirty days, I was healthier. I'd lost thirteen pounds, my skin was clearing, and I had more money in the bank— all that cash I'd saved from not drinking. I even started waking up early to work out. The positive changes were encouraging enough that I decided to keep going and see where it would take me.

Around the sixty-day mark, I occasionally craved a glass of red wine with dinner or a Bombay Sapphire and tonic at the end of the workday. When it was hot outside, I couldn't help but think, *I could smash a cold beer right now.* But I trained myself to breathe deeply, down a tall glass of water, and simply allow the feeling to pass. And it did pass.

After three months, I turned the corner and was developing power over alcohol. I felt terrific. I had a natural energy I hadn't known since I was much younger. I was getting compliments on my improved looks. And despite not drinking, I still managed to have wildly entertaining nights out—even with friends and colleagues drinking heavily around me.

Back then, I was single. To my surprise, my dating life actually improved without booze. My conversations with women became much more meaningful, and my dates were impressed by my self-discipline and commitment to my health.

By month six, I was in the zone. I was generating a consistent seven to eight hours of good sleep a night, as my body settled into its natural circadian rhythm. I could go out with people drinking around me and still have fun, or I could stay in and not even think about alcohol. I was up early in the morning to exercise, shower, and have breakfast, and I was ready to tackle the day by the time friends and colleagues were slowly waking up from a night of after-work cocktails and disrupted sleep.

By the time I approached one year without alcohol, I noticed the dramatic and lasting changes that would truly reshape my life. My relationships—with family, romantic partners, colleagues, and clients—were considerably improved. I thought more about how I could help others than how they could help me. I was more relaxed and made better decisions. My productivity soared and new opportunities came my way, including becoming an anchor on ESPN's *SportsCenter* and finding a personal mentor in

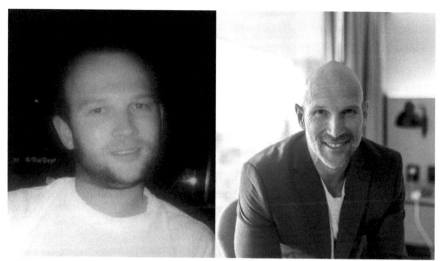

I was tired, inflamed, and flabby for much of my twenties and thirties while drinking. Now, at forty-nine, I'm alcohol-free and in the best shape of my life.

entrepreneur Tai Lopez. Clear in body and mind, I had the energy, discipline, and motivation to excel at ESPN and then to start two businesses of my own.

When I reached the milestone of one year without drinking, I found myself at a pub in Austin, again during South by Southwest. To celebrate a year of alcohol-free living, I did something counter-intuitive: I ordered a Budweiser in a pub and put it to my mouth. It smelled good. I had every intention of drinking that beer, but something stopped me. I paused for a minute and considered how my life had transformed. The pros of an alcohol-free life had proved to far outweigh the cons. I put the Budweiser down, and I haven't so much as picked up a drink since. Not drinking transformed me—personally and professionally. I believe it will transform you, too.

WHY GO ALCOHOL-FREE?

From a professional standpoint, going alcohol-free is a great strategy for business and career improvement. It's a lifestyle that allows you to harness the full force of your energy and focus on delivering meaningful results. However, I have a feeling that professional achievement is not the real reason you're picking up this book. My guess is that you're the type of person who'd likely be successful, whether you're drinking or not, because you probably already have been. In fact, the majority of our clients have a high level of professional standing in their careers before they begin working with us to become alcohol-free.

You are an intelligent person. You know that drinking isn't good for you—but that's not enough to make you stop. The biggest reason people keep drinking, even when they don't really want to, is fear. They are afraid of the unknown and afraid of their identity changing if they quit drinking. They are afraid of being dull and boring at social events. They are afraid that if they try to quit and slip later, then they must really be broken. To avoid that happening, they find it easier to just continue drinking. The fear of not succeeding prevents them from trying in the first place. It's backwards logic. They don't like drinking and the consequences it brings, but at least they know what life looks like in the comfort zone.

One member of our *Project 90* coaching program reflected on their decision to join the program, sharing: "I've been stuck in a rut, feeling unmotivated and foggy. I want to feel better, sleep better, and rebuild better relationships with my kids and employees." Sound familiar?

Maybe you've been drifting for years. You've been existing, but not fully engaged with your family, career or personal life. Alcohol is keeping you stuck in a loop. Waking up every day, doing the same thing. Aren't you sick of feeling the same tired body, foggy and hazy emotions from another night of drinking?

Maybe your relationships are hurting deeply. Some of our clients have children or grandchildren who no longer take their calls because of the damage done by years of alcohol-infused parenting. Clients admit to us that they have missed showing up for friends, family and spouses because of their alcohol habit—and now their most important relationships are in serious trouble from decades of neglect.

Many have tried AA or even in-patient rehab before, but they don't want to deal with the time, expense and stigma of something so intense only for it to fail again. Oftentimes, our clients will initially be embarrassed to even tell family or friends that they're inside of a community of people who are trying to quit drinking. They're embarrassed about what others would think of them. All of them want to be better parents, grandparents and partners. And they want to be better to themselves, too.

These are just a few of the many reasons why our clients embrace the alcohol-free lifestyle.

I want you to know that this is your chance to make a generational impact on your family. You may come from a long line of men and women who had serious problems with alcohol. You may be the unwilling recipient of a lot of bad habits and trauma, passed down to you by people whose lives were torn apart by alcohol. By reading and applying the information in this book, you are now taking control of your own lineage by deciding that those habits stop with you. Implementing what you'll learn in these pages may be the single most significant contribution you can make to everyone who comes after you.

No matter how bad your relationship with alcohol currently is, you can change it—not with will power and wishful thinking, but with a proven, science-based method for quitting alcohol based on over a decade's worth of our own research that has already helped thousands of people. You can become alcohol-free and reap all the rewards of a life no longer weighed down by the burden of drinking.

On the other hand, you don't need to hit rock bottom to begin the climb back to the top. You can start the transformation here and now. Just imagine how your health, wealth, love, and happiness would change if you reclaimed the energy you currently direct toward drinking. Imagine the relationships you could repair if alcohol wasn't in the way.

HOW TO USE THIS BOOK

CLEAR is the blueprint for the high performer who knows that alcohol isn't supporting their ability to live, work, and create at their highest capacity. This includes small business owners, multimillion-dollar entrepreneurs, CEOs, executives, professionals, career-focused employees, creatives, and athletes who are ready to take their power back from a long-term drinking habit. It's for the natural achiever who knows they want to change their relationship with alcohol, but needs a step-by-step system to walk them through the process from A to Z.

You might notice that I made this book a bit shorter than typical self-help books. When I read books looking to solve a specific problem and I find the author repeating themselves over and over again, I get annoyed. I learned to speed read years ago to help solve this problem when downloading new information into my brain, but I appreciate brevity all the same. I'm used to working with people who want their personal development in a hurry, so you'll find this book is straight to the point. You can read the whole thing in a weekend and get to work transforming your life by Monday.

In Part I of this book, we'll challenge your beliefs around alcohol and help you rewrite the story you've been telling yourself about drinking.

In Part II, we'll break down the facts about how alcohol (even in small amounts) can negatively impact your health, performance, success, and happiness—and, in turn, how giving it up naturally and effortlessly will enhance each of these areas of your life.

In Part III, you'll find a guide to getting started on your own journey to live an alcohol-free lifestyle—including dealing with all the inevitable challenges that will arise on the way to lasting change.

At the end of each chapter, you'll also find:

> » A summary of key takeaways from the chapter for quick review.

» Reflections you can utilize to begin getting clarity and making progress immediately.

» Real stories from members of the Alcohol-Free Lifestyle community who have successfully overcome the challenges you're going through.

» An opportunity to connect with an Alcohol-Free Lifestyle coach. If at any time while reading this book, you're ready to get support from a professional on our team to help you quit drinking for good, you can register for a free call by going to www.alcoholfreelifestyle.com/resources.

Quitting alcohol is a secret weapon for peak performers striving to unlock their potential. I've seen my clients make more money, have more fun, feel more at ease, and tell me that they love their life more when alcohol is no longer a part of it.

I have seen clients save their marriage, be more present with their children, heal their relationships, finally accomplish "bucket list" items, and feel a sense of immense joy when alcohol is no longer a roadblock.

Now, it's your turn.

JAMES SWANWICK
CEO | Alcohol-Free Lifestyle

PART I

REWRITING YOUR STORY ABOUT ALCOHOL

CHAPTER 1:

WHY WE DRINK

*"Drunkenness is nothing
but voluntary madness."*

—SENECA

I F YOU HAD A FRIEND who constantly talked about you behind your back...

Who took every opportunity to slow you down and clearly didn't have your best interests in mind...

Would you still continue spending time with them? Better yet: Would you let this friend come over two or three times a week and poison you? Of course not. Only a crazy person or someone who doesn't value their life would do something like that.

Yet that's exactly what you're doing with alcohol. Alcohol is that friend talking behind your back, that slithering snake in the grass sabotaging your progress and killing you a little bit every day. This book is all about how you can learn to take the power back from alcohol and redefine the relationship you have with it forever.

THIS BOOK IS NOT FOR "ALCOHOLICS"

You're not an alcoholic. The image society has painted of alcoholics is people who are down and out, who have lost everything and are living in alleys. In television and in movies, the alcoholic is often portrayed as a loser who is sick without alcohol and totally out of control.

That's not you. In fact, you're the exact opposite of that stereotype, which is why you've probably never identified with the term alcoholic. To many, that word feels derogatory and extreme. However, just because you're functioning at a high level while still including alcohol in your life doesn't mean that you're not experiencing the negative side effects and addictive qualities of drinking.

You have superpowers, but you're blocking them with booze.

All of my clients at our stop-drinking coaching organization, Alcohol-Free Lifestyle, are high performers who consider themselves top tier at what they do. They are business owners, executives, and professionals in high-stakes careers who are used to being successful at work—but deep down, they are often lacking in personal fulfillment and connection. Most of them express a desire to heal their relationships and be more present with their family and friends. They suspect that quitting alcohol might help them reach a new level of enjoyment in life—and they're right.

Simply add up all the hours you think about drinking, going to other locations to drink, consuming the drinks, then recuperating from drinking. You'll find enough energy being wasted in pursuit of alcohol to change your life when properly redirected.

People with AUD are often considered casual drinkers by normal standards. They may have just a few drinks, a few nights per week. Those with mild to moderate AUD aren't blacking out, driving drunk, or making dumb decisions. They likely have demanding careers and loving families whom they regularly show up for—but in the back of their minds, many of them, like you, probably know that drinking is dulling their edge. It's a source of energetic drain that's stopping them from being at full capacity, even if others don't notice it.

For the purposes of this book, we'll use the term *alcohol use disorder* (or AUD) to describe what has been called alcoholism in the past—though there may be quotes from older sources that use more outdated language. Don't get hung up on the terminology too much. The sentiment is the same. Smart people have known for thousands of years that alcohol makes you dumber.

This book is designed to help you find your edge again and exceed your own expectations of what's possible. You just have to learn how to reverse engineer the habit loop you have with alcohol. Before we get to that, it's useful to understand exactly why you feel so drawn to drinking in the first place.

HUMANS + ALCOHOL: AN ANCIENT KINSHIP

The relationship between humans and alcohol is thousands of years old. We see evidence of the power of alcohol in ancient rituals and celebrations all the way to modern day. You'll find a bottle of booze on every page of the history of human existence.

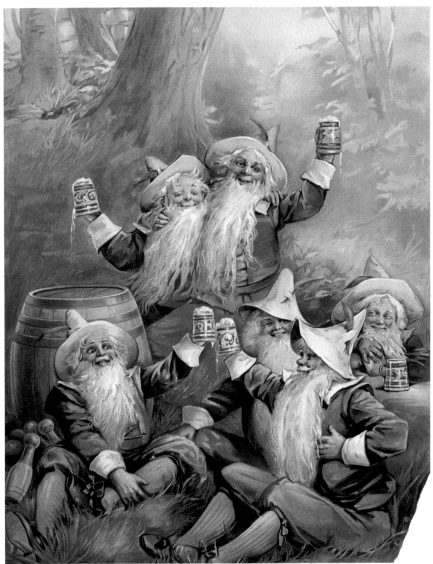

Humanity's relationship with alcohol has always had a mythical component. This German beer advertisement from 1898 features happy, drunk gnomes.

Alcoholic beverages have long been known for their medicinal and pain-killing properties. Many cultures of the past have actually considered it healthy to consume. Wine played a central role in the diets of both the Greek and Roman empires—and in the Middle Ages, the monks brewed beer because it was actually safer to drink than water, which was often contaminated. Not a bad reason to be drunk, I guess.

Human social dynamics around drinking can be tricky. Alcohol has traditionally been associated with good times, social standing, and has generally been seen as a sign of hospitality. Drinking is something you do out of camaraderie, which makes it hard for many people to reject a drink without feeling that they are jeopardizing the friendship itself. In some cultures, refusing a drink can be seen as disrespectful. There's a lot of peer pressure around drinking, even at the professional level.

Any family gathering, birthday party, wedding, or important family dinner is likely to have alcohol involved. Even at parties for their children, many parents are likely to be drinking. When everybody around you is drinking and having a good time, it feels like refusing would make it harder to have fun. It can make you feel left out.

At work, many after-hours functions may revolve around alcohol. This reinforces the notion that drinking is a required part of building rapport, closing sales, or getting promoted. This perception is false, but the idea still creates a strong incentive to order another shot.

If you're an executive, sales leader, consultant, or professional, you have probably felt compelled to have a drink with a client at some point in order to close the deal—even if you didn't really want

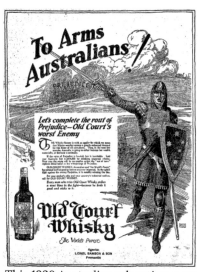

This 1928 Australian advertisement for Old Court Whisky evokes masculinity, ancient archetypes and the call to power. Exaggerate much?

to. There's no shame in it. We've all given in to the temptation to put on a song and dance when we want to impress someone.

Now, answer these questions truthfully: Do you think the conversation would have been easier if you had your brain's full horsepower available to you? Do you think you would have had a better chance if you were completely sharp and focused during the conversation?

Before joining the Alcohol-Free Lifestyle, many of my clients found it challenging to refuse drinks offered by colleagues and potential clients, fearing it could potentially hinder their career prospects. They were worried that people would think they're no fun, so they drank even when they didn't want to. This paradox is a reality for many top performers.

The perception that alcohol is an important and necessary component of social interaction has been programmed into your subconscious through culture and reinforced by the multibillion-dollar conglomerate of companies known as Big Alcohol.

Today, it's time to see through the façade and understand the games that are being played all around us.

HOW BIG ALCOHOL TRICKS CONSUMERS INTO DRINKING

French scientist Serge Renaud became a hero of the wine industry in 1991 when he announced on the American TV news show 60 Minutes that drinking red wine was good for the heart. 60 Minutes journalist Morley Safer latched onto the claim. He raised a glass of red wine with a smile to the 33 million viewers who tuned in that night. The day following the episode, all U.S. airlines reportedly ran out of red wine, and red wine sales began to skyrocket.

For the next month, wine sales in the U.S. spiked by 44 percent. That's two and a half million bottles. When the episode was re-aired in 1992, they spiked again, by 49 percent. Sales of red wine for the entire year were up by a total of 39 percent. Americans never looked back, devouring more Merlot, Malbec and Cabernet every year—as if it was protecting them from death and somehow improving their health.

There was just one big problem: the claim that alcohol is good for your health has now been shown to be completely and utterly false. A 2022 study[4] of 35,000 middle-aged adults showed that even one seemingly innocent drink a night was enough to cause some level of damage to vital organs.

Despite these findings, Big Alcohol often funds so-called "health studies" on alcohol in a bid to legitimize daily drinking and protect its profits. These multibillion-dollar companies are doing everything they can to suppress scientific proof that even small amounts of alcohol are bad for you. All they care about is profit.

In fact, a 2023 meta-study by Professor Tim Stockwell of the University of Victoria uncovered what he refers to as a "significant bias" in health studies by authors with ties to the alcohol industry. Professor Stockwell conducted a study of 107 previously published papers on alcohol involving nearly 5 million participants over forty years.

His research revealed that studies claiming a glass of red wine was good for heart health were either skewed and or biased towards alcohol companies. This is in line with tactics Big Alcohol has used for decades to fool consumers. In the 1960s, major beer companies collaborated with alcohol researchers, including Thomas Turner—a former dean of John Hopkins University Medical School—to create what's now called the Foundation for Alcohol Research. This foundation has gone on to fund more than 500 studies and awarded grants to universities and researchers, using their money to exert influence over the studies.

For example, a *New York Times* article revealed that the National Institute on Alcohol Abuse and Alcoholism had allowed alcohol company leaders to review the study's design and vet principle investigators before the trial even started. The institute even assured an alcohol industry group that the trial would show that moderate drinking was safe. Ultimately, the trial failed to begin because of outrage at the ethical lines being crossed.

This type of heavy-handed effort to bias science needs to be exposed.

HOW HOLLYWOOD FALSELY GLAMORIZES ALCOHOL

Movies, television, and commercials paint alcohol as glamorous, fun, and essential parts of a life well-lived. Whether it's James Bond sipping his signature "shaken, not stirred" martini in bar, an ad that shows a group of frat friends laughing over cases of Coors, or a television show that highlights a gigantic glass of wine the main character drinks every night after work—you are being programmed to think you need alcohol to be cool, sophisticated, or fun.

Brands like Budweiser and Corona have perfected the narrative of carefree time with friends and family being centered around beer. They love to show scenic beaches, colorful cities, or fun events to sell the idea that their product is essential for having a good time. These images are designed to evoke a sense of FOMO (fear of missing out). But don't worry; you're not missing anything. Because it's not reality. It's just marketing.

In TV series like *Mad Men*, characters are always drinking whiskey in posh settings, dressed in immaculate wardrobe, sipping out of beautiful crystal. This type of depiction shapes your perception of alcohol as stylish. And it's intentional.

Alcohol is often attached to other symbols of power like sex and money. That's why the alcohol industry spends billions of dollars annually on advertising that glorifies and promotes drinking—because it works. These advertisements feature the most attractive people they can find, paired with the best music and the hottest visuals they can create.

This marketing strategy can trick your brain into creating a powerful association between alcohol and success, despite the

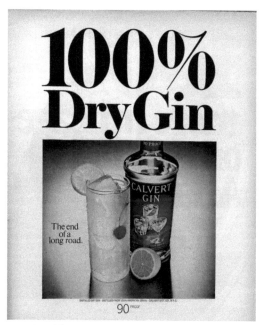

This 1960's Calvert Gin ad has the "Mad Men" era feeling to it. It communicates the
idea that drinking is cool, refreshing and necessary after a hard day at work.

fact that based on mounting research, alcohol consumption actually has a negative effect on overall happiness and success.

"Habit-forming products align with the user's daily routines
and emotions," says former Stanford lecturer and author Nir Eyal
in his book *Hooked: How to Build Habit-Forming Products*.[5] He
adds:

> *An internal trigger is an itch that comes from a feeling or
> emotion. For example, feeling lonely might trigger one to
> check Facebook. The user's brain is cued to check it for relief.
> Habit-forming products solve a pain point by creating an
> association with the user's internal triggers. Subsequently,
> users show up repeatedly, without any external prompt.*

Much of this habit-forming and brainwashing begins before we
are old enough to recognize it or fight it off. Thus, it comes as no
surprise that studies have shown exposure to alcohol advertising

Why Most People Drink

Whether it's stress, social pressure or just a bad habit, most people have more than one reason they drink alcohol. What are yours?

increases the likelihood of underage drinking. This is because young people are particularly susceptible to marketing messages that insinuate alcohol is necessary to fit in with their peers. Most people carry this belief through school into their working life without ever reexamining whether it's true or not.

You have permission to question your beliefs, even if you've had them for your entire life. Let me ask you a potentially sensitive question: When was the last time you seriously examined your relationship with alcohol?

UNPACKING THE PSYCHOLOGICAL FACTORS BEHIND ALCOHOL CONSUMPTION

The number one reason most people drink is to cope with stress. Getting drunk temporarily relaxes you. I know that's what it did for me. You feel stressed, so, naturally, you want to relieve that stress—and the only way you know how to do that is to drink alcohol. The ugly truth is, alcohol doesn't relieve stress. It actually creates more stress.

Here's a perspective shift: when you drink, you're not actually drinking for pleasure. You think you're enjoying a nice glass of wine, but the wine isn't what you're after. In reality, you're drinking to relieve yourself of your alcohol withdrawal.

Alcohol is a highly addictive drug and that means it creates intense cravings and withdrawal symptoms. It always leaves you wanting more. As soon as the first drop hits your lips, the game is on. Your brain thinks that the only way to relieve the discomfort of alcohol cravings is to drink more alcohol. The more you drink, the more pronounced the cravings become. Lost in the cycle of craving and the illusion of relief, you think you're solving the original problem of stress with a beer—but all you're really doing is putting on weight, disrupting your sleep, and feeling crappy in the morning.

It's time to get off the train. It's not headed towards the relief you're searching for—and never will. Alcohol offers you a sense of momentary relief from the anxiety and tension of being a top performer. For many professionals, it becomes the go-to solution after a tough day as a way to unwind. You love alcohol because it can numb you for a bit. It can help you forget about the severity of your problems for a few hours. The problem is that outside of immediate pain relief, it can also cause a lot of additional stress and anxiety over time.

After a while, the stress that drinking causes you will outweigh the short-term benefits you get from consuming it. You just need to be honest with yourself about whether or not you've reached that point. If so, now is a great time to make a new decision.

Consider the example of a high-powered attorney who works long hours and deals with constant pressure all the time. At the end of the day, she pours herself a glass of wine to unwind. Harmless, right? Wrong. It starts off as one glass. Then it turns into two or three. Eventually what started as a one-off way to relax becomes a nightly ritual. Over time, this unhealthy cycle begins to leak into her personal health, her performance at work, and her marriage. The negative impact of alcohol over a period of years is gradual, but can be astounding in scope. Not worth it.

Over time, your brain starts to associate alcohol with pleasure and relaxation, reinforcing the behavior to drink. It might start as a drink with dinner or a few beers on the weekend. As the habit becomes more deeply ingrained, you start to drink more and more. As you press that pleasure button repeatedly, the brain releases dopamine in response. You begin to crave the stimulation provided by the response your brain provides to alcohol. This craving leads to increased consumption and, eventually, addiction.

This is the habit loop. Around and around we go.

As the book progresses, we'll dive deeper into the science of habit formation. For now, let's just cover the basics. Habits are formed through a cycle known as the habit loop, a term originally coined by author Charles Duhigg in his book *The Power of Habit*.

The habit loop, says Duhigg, consists of three components[6]: the cue, the routine, and the reward. This cycle plays a significant role in the development of alcohol habits.

> » **Cue:** This is the trigger that initiates the habit. That might include social events, seeing others drink, or specific times of day (like after work). It could also include emotional states, such as feeling stressed.
> » **Routine:** This is the behavior itself—in this case, consuming alcohol. When faced with the cue (e.g., stress), the individual engages in the routine (drinking) to address the cue.
> » **Reward:** This is the positive reinforcement that follows the routine, reinforcing the habit loop. Alcohol provides a temporary sense of pleasure, relaxation, or escape from negative emotions.

This loop is the reason why you can't stop drinking, even when you want to. The elephant in the room here is dopamine, the neurotransmitter associated with pleasure and reward.

THE ROLE OF DOPAMINE

When you drink, dopamine is released and you feel euphoric. This reinforces the habit loop. Sex, drugs, and alcohol all release dopamine. We love dopamine so much, we'll do whatever we can to get more of that feeling—even if the behavior is detrimental to our health.

The release of dopamine reinforces whatever behavior the brain associates with releasing it. That makes you more likely to do the things which reliably release dopamine. The more you drink, the more your brain becomes conditioned to expect a surge of dopamine with each drink. This expectation creates a craving, and the craving drives your behavior to drink in order to satisfy the craving. Over time, the brain requires more alcohol to achieve the same dopamine response, leading to increased consumption and tolerance.

Drinking changes the brain's structure and function. When you drink alcohol, you can damage your brain cells, slow your cognition, and alter the brain's chemistry. The prefrontal cortex, which is responsible for decision-making, impulse control, and rational thought, can be particularly affected. The 2022 study of 35,000 middle-aged adults I referenced earlier found that damage to the brain begins with just one or two drinks per day and becomes significantly worse as alcohol intake increases.

This is why it's so difficult for you to resist cravings and make healthy decisions sometimes. You're fighting a deeply embedded habit with a partially broken brain. A little bit dramatic, yes. But if you've ever tried to break your alcohol habit loop and failed over and over again, you know it's true. It's an elegant, deadly treadmill.

The only way to save your body and your mind from the inevitable effects of alcohol is to get off the treadmill as quickly as possible—and never look back. Since you're still very early in your journey to become alcohol-free, you might as well get a crystal clear picture of what you're up against.

I wanted to add something I feel is important here regarding your approach to quitting drinking: although many of our successful members never look at a drink the same way again, you may never get to a point where a nice glass of wine with dinner doesn't sound good.

You may still know that a cold beer on a hot afternoon would be enjoyable. That's completely normal, and it's to be expected. The difference is, after reading this book, you'll most likely recognize that enjoying something isn't reason enough to continue doing it—especially considering the toll that alcohol has taken on the health of your body, mind and relationships.

Let's look at exactly how alcohol affects your body first.

HOW ALCOHOL DESTROYS YOUR BODY FROM THE INSIDE

In a recent coaching conversation, a *Project 90* client expressed to me that the reason for joining was to finally take control of their drinking, saying: "I drink daily—five to six glasses of wine—and my physical cravings have taken over. It's just a matter of time before I lose my physical health, my partner, and my job."

That awareness is the first step in making positive change.

The habit loop with alcohol has major physical consequences. There's no simpler way to say it: alcohol trashes your body. Instead of looking at alcohol longingly as something to be enjoyed, begin to see it as what it really is: attractively packaged poison. This might sound a little harsh, but it's also a wake-up call.

When you drink, every major organ pays the price. Though it feels good in the moment, drinking can damage your liver, heart, and pancreas, increase your risk of cancer, and weaken your immune system. Excessive drinking can also lead to neurological problems, such as memory loss and cognitive decline. If anyone in your family has severe alcohol use disorder, you've seen the impact that a lifetime of drinking has on a person.

Here are some of the ways that alcohol consumption—even in small or moderate amounts—negatively impacts your body. If it sounds like a laundry list, that's because it is.

ALCOHOL DAMAGES YOUR LIVER

You probably already know that alcohol damages your liver. But do you know what impact that can have on your day-to-day health? A damaged liver can cause clogging in your detoxification pathways, which can contribute to chronic disease.[7]

The liver is responsible for metabolizing alcohol, but it can easily become overwhelmed by excessive drinking. Conditions such as fatty liver, alcoholic hepatitis, fibrosis, and cirrhosis are common among heavy drinkers.[8]

» **Fatty liver:** This condition occurs when fat builds up in the liver cells.
» **Alcoholic hepatitis:** Inflammation of the liver caused by heavy drinking.
» **Fibrosis and cirrhosis:** Long-term drinking can cause scar tissue to form in the liver (fibrosis), which can progress to cirrhosis, a severe and often irreversible condition that impairs liver function.

And you don't need to be a serious alcoholic to experience the devastating effects. Research shows that liver disease has risen in the UK by a staggering 400 percent since the 1970s.

"Those at risk are not just chronic alcohol abusers, but also middle-aged professionals who drink a little too much most nights,"[9] says Dr. Debbie Shawcross at King's College Hospital Liver Unit. No such study appears to have been done in Americans, though it's reasonable to assume a similar trend is happening here.

ALCOHOL INCREASES YOUR RISK OF HIGH BLOOD PRESSURE, STROKE, AND HEART PROBLEMS

One *Project 90* client opened up about why they'd finally reached a breaking point with alcohol, confessing: "I've been drinking daily—beer and vodka—from 5:30 p.m. to 11 p.m. My blood pressure is high, and I feel like I'm slowly killing myself."

But it doesn't have to be this way.

Alcohol consumption is strongly linked to high blood pressure (hypertension) due to its effects on the cardiovascular system.[10] When consumed in excessive amounts, alcohol can cause an increase in heart rate and trigger the release of stress hormones, which constrict blood vessels.

This narrowing of the blood vessels forces the heart to pump harder, resulting in elevated blood pressure. Even moderate drinking, especially if done regularly, has been associated with higher systolic and diastolic blood pressure levels, according to multiple studies.[11] We all had an aunt who told us a glass of wine every day was good for your heart. It turns out that she was wrong—and her advice may have been deadly.

Case in point: in addition to stressing the heart, alcohol also impacts the heart's structure and functionality, particularly in cases of alcoholic cardiomyopathy. This condition involves a weakening of the heart muscle due to drinking. When this happens, the heart becomes unable to pump blood effectively and you're in danger of heart failure.

Alcohol's role in increasing the risk of stroke cannot be overstated, either. According to recent research at the University of Cambridge,[12] both ischemic and hemorrhagic strokes, which result from blocked or ruptured blood vessels in the brain, respectively, are more likely with heavy alcohol consumption. This is due to alcohol's contribution to atherosclerosis, a critical factor in stroke occurrence, highlighting another severe risk factor associated with drinking.

Repeat after me: "I'll take a club soda with lime, thanks."

ALCOHOL INCREASES YOUR RISK OF
DIABETES BY DAMAGING YOUR PANCREAS

The pancreas plays a critical role in both digestion and blood sugar regulation by producing enzymes that aid digestion. Chronic alcohol consumption leads to the activation of digestive enzymes while they're still inside the pancreas, causing irritation and inflammation called pancreatitis. This premature activation is harmful because it starts digesting the pancreas itself.

Chronic pancreatitis can further exacerbate insulin resistance, which means your body will require more insulin to manage blood glucose levels. This stress on the pancreas can hinder its capacity to function properly, significantly increasing your risk of developing type 2 diabetes. It's all connected.

According to the International Diabetes Federation,[13] approximately 6.7 million deaths in 2021 were attributed to diabetes, accounting for around 12.2 percent of all global mortality.

Diabetes is a silent killer, delivered to a willing population through the vehicle of alcohol.

ALCOHOL SIGNIFICANTLY
INCREASES YOUR CANCER RISK

Did you know that alcohol has been classified as a Group 1 carcinogen by the International Agency for Research on Cancer (IARC)? Everybody is terrified of getting cancer. Alcohol causes cancer, yet so many smart people still drink. What's wrong with this picture? I guess even top performers still need convincing that booze is as bad for us as research says it is.

Rest assured, this classification is based on strong evidence linking alcohol consumption to various cancers. A few with the highest correlation to alcohol consumption include:

» Mouth, throat, and esophageal cancer[14]
» Liver cancer

» Breast cancer[15]
» Colorectal cancer

The carcinogenicity is largely due to ethanol, the active ingre-
dient in alcoholic beverages, which metabolizes into acetaldehyde,
a compound that damages DNA and other cellular structures,
leading to disease.[16]

The dose-response relationship between alcohol consumption
and cancer risk is particularly alarming. This relationship suggests
that even moderate levels of drinking, often perceived as safe,
incrementally increase the risk of developing various cancers.
Such findings are crucial in understanding why alcohol is grouped
with notorious carcinogens like tobacco and asbestos. When it
comes to alcohol and cancer, no amount is conclusively safe.

ALCOHOL CAUSES BRAIN DAMAGE AND DEPRESSION

Though we'll discuss this topic in much greater detail later in the
book, it's worth noting here that chronic alcohol consumption
can lead to a range of neurological issues, affecting both mental
and physical health. Those issues include:

» **Memory loss and cognitive decline[17]:** Long-term drinking
  can lead to memory loss and an increased risk of dementia.
» **Neuropathy:** Damage to the peripheral nerves (neuropathy) as a result of drinking can cause pain, tingling, and
  weakness in the extremities.
» **Brain damage:** Prolonged alcohol use can cause physical
  changes in your brain, affecting areas responsible for coordination, balance, and decision-making.

In addition to the physical effects on the brain, chronic alcohol
consumption can exacerbate mental health issues like anxiety

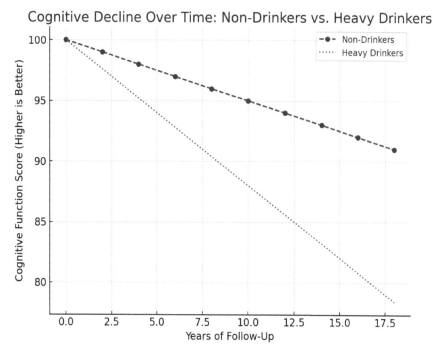

This graph highlights how chronic heavy alcohol consumption accelerates cognitive deterioration compared to abstaining from alcohol.

and depression. According to Yale researchers in 1998,[18] four large community-based epidemiological studies (n = 22,000) in Europe and the USA "consistently demonstrated a two-to-three-fold increase in the lifetime prevalence of anxiety and depression in those with DSM–III or DSM–III–R alcohol abuse or dependence."

A *Project 90* member recently revealed: "I've been drinking wine nightly for years. My anxiety wakes me up, and I think about drinking just to cope. It's a cycle I want to break to find peace and ease in my life." Going alcohol-free is how they finally found relief.

If you're someone who already struggles with anxiety and depression, alcohol can make them both much worse. If you've never dealt with these problems before, alcohol can create them. As a top performer, your number one asset is your mind. You need every shred of advantage you can muster on the competitive landscapes of business and life. Dropping alcohol is a no-brainer.

ALCOHOL CREATES GASTROINTESTINAL, IMMUNE SYSTEM, AND NUTRIENT ABSORPTION PROBLEMS

Ever experienced severe heartburn after a night of drinking? This is a direct result of alcohol irritating your stomach lining and increasing acidity. Drinking is a major culprit in causing leaky gut syndrome—a condition where the lining of the small intestine becomes damaged, allowing undigested food particles, toxic waste products, and bacteria to "leak" through the intestines into the bloodstream.

Leaky gut syndrome can have an enormous impact on our immune function and overall health and well-being. Just one night of bingeing increases your gut permeability, according to multiple studies.[19] When harmful toxins and bacteria leak from your digestive system into your bloodstream, it prompts an immune-system response that can eventually lead to liver disease and other health problems. Every time you drink, you are potentially weakening the lining of your intestines.

Regular drinking not only increases the risk of developing stomach ulcers but also significantly hampers the body's ability to absorb essential nutrients. Drinking depletes the body of vitamins like folate and minerals such as magnesium, both crucial for maintaining cellular and metabolic health. This malabsorption can lead to deficiencies that affect various bodily functions, including nerve function, blood cell production, and bone health.[20]

ALCOHOL CAUSES AND EXACERBATES SKIN DISEASES

Ever looked in the mirror after a night of heavy drinking? I'm guessing you don't feel too flattered with what you see. That's because alcohol wreaks havoc on your skin—which just happens to be your biggest organ.

Drinking leads to dry skin, flakiness, puffiness around the eyes, and premature wrinkles. It also dilates your blood vessels, giving you a red and blotchy complexion.[21] The excess sugars (especially with beer and wine) damage the DNA and collagen in your skin. Alcohol also impairs the body's ability to absorb vital antioxidants and vitamins, such as vitamin A, which is crucial for skin renewal and moisture retention. This nutritional deficiency exacerbates skin damage and makes you look older.

And that's not all: A 2023 paper titled "Advances in Relationship Between Alcohol Consumption and Skin Diseases"[22] showed that alcohol can both cause and exacerbate existing skin diseases, including rosacea, psoriasis, and even skin cancer.

Apparently, the fountain of youth is not at the bottom of the wine bottle.

ALCOHOL CAUSES SEXUAL AND REPRODUCTIVE HEALTH ISSUES

Gentlemen, think about a time when you had a few too many drinks on a date night. Initially, the alcohol might have made you feel more confident and relaxed, but when it came time to perform, you found it, say, challenging.

A 2021 study that evaluated the association between alcohol consumption and risk of erectile dysfunction (ED) found that "if taken chronically, it could provoke vascular damages."[23]

It's called "whiskey dick" for a reason, my friend.

This is because alcohol depresses nerve centers in the hypothalamus that control sexual arousal and performance. Although you may feel hornier after a few drinks, sexual performance has been shown to decrease in both the short-term and long-term.

Almost three-quarters of men with alcohol dependence have at least one sexual health issue, such as low desire, erectile dysfunction, or premature ejaculation, according to numerous studies.[24]

Ladies don't get off easy, either.

Consider a professional woman who enjoys social drinking with friends a few times a week. Harmless fun, right? While it may seem like a normal part of her social routine, frequent alcohol consumption can disrupt her hormonal balance, leading to irregular menstrual cycles and potential fertility issues.[25] Drinking during pregnancy can cause fetal alcohol syndrome, leading to developmental issues and lifelong disabilities in the child.

Alcohol also elevates her risk of breast cancer significantly. One prominent study showed "a risk relationship between alcohol consumption and the risk of breast cancer, even at low levels of consumption. Due to this strong relationship, and to the amount of alcohol consumed globally, the incidence of and mortality from alcohol-attributable breast cancer is large."[26]

* * *

It's true that the "casual drinker" may not experience some of the more extreme consequences listed above. However, it would be inaccurate to say that alcohol is having a neutral or positive effect on the body. The problems listed above are not "side effects" of alcohol, they are direct effects that can happen on a sliding scale to anybody who consumes alcohol.

According to a report from the CDC:

> "From 2018 to 2021, there was a nearly 23% increase in deaths attributed to excessive alcohol use. This increase is particularly alarming and has been linked to greater alcohol availability and changes in alcohol policy during the COVID-19 pandemic."[27]

If you want to be the absolute best in your field, you have to use your mind, body and spirit to generate energy. Why would you flirt with any substance that lowers your energy and robs you of the opportunity to perform at the highest level?

Why would you want to risk any of these draining and potentially deadly direct effects just to participate in a social custom that, upon closer examination, you probably don't even enjoy that much anyway?

The answers to those questions aren't logical. They are emotional—and that's the reason why it is so hard to stop drinking, even when you want to. But what about just "cutting back" on booze a little bit?

Here's why I think the idea of "moderation" is a slippery slope.

WHAT ABOUT DRINKING IN MODERATION?

No book on quitting alcohol would be complete without playing devil's advocate at least once. What most people really want to know is, "Why can't I just drink a little bit? The Greeks said, 'Everything in moderation,' right?"

The answer is: Yes, having less is always better. If you're currently having ten drinks every time you go out with your friends, and after reading this book you reduce that number to three, you'll still experience a tremendous benefit, and I'd consider that a win. Ultimately, my goal is to use logic, emotion, research, and case studies to persuade you to drop your number to zero and live an alcohol-free lifestyle.

For instance, a fascinating 2012 study from Scotland ranked nineteen commonly used drugs on the relative harm of drug misuse to self and others. They reported:

> Heroin, crack cocaine, crystal meth, alcohol and cocaine were in the top five places for all categories of harm... There was no stepped categorical distinction in harm between the different legal and illegal substances. Heroin was viewed as the most harmful, and cannabis the least harmful of the substances studied. Alcohol was ranked as the fourth most harmful substance, with alcohol, nicotine and volatile solvents being viewed as more harmful than some class A drugs.[28]

The results from the study are reproduced in table 1.1.

Of nineteen drugs listed, alcohol was ranked as the fourth most harmful—yet it's available legally in unlimited quantities on every street corner. A 2020 study from Germany corroborated these findings.

SUBSTANCE	PERSONAL HARM SCORE	SOCIAL HARM SCORE	TOTAL SCORE
HEROIN	2.76	2.72	2.74
CRACK COCAINE	2.74	2.60	2.69
CRYSTAL METH	2.69	2.54	2.63
ALCOHOL	2.55	2.70	2.56
COCAINE	2.54	2.33	2.46
INHALED SOLVENTS	2.38	2.18	2.31
NICOTINE	2.42	2.23	2.29
BENZOS	2.33	2.17	2.27
KETAMINE	2.24	1.97	2.13
BARBITURATES	2.25	1.91	2.12
AMPHETAMINES	2.24	1.89	2.11
METHADONE	2.19	1.96	2.10
CODEINE	2.05	1.89	1.98
BUPRENORPHINE	2.04	1.83	1.96
LSD	2.04	1.87	1.95
ECSTASY	2.07	1.74	1.92
RITALIN	1.86	1.62	1.74
MAGIC MUSHROOMS	1.88	1.60	1.74
CANNABIS	1.86	1.61	1.73

Table 1.1

HARMS TO USERS	HARMS TO OTHERS
DRUG-SPECIFIC MORTALITY	INJURY
DRUG-RELATED MORTALITY	CRIME
DRUG-SPECIFIC HARM	ECONOMIC COST
DRUG-RELATED HARM	IMPACT ON FAMILY LIFE
DEPENDENCE	INTERNATIONAL DAMAGE
DRUG-SPECIFIC IMPAIRMENT OF MENTAL FUNCTIONING	ENVIRONMENTAL DAMAGE
DRUG-RELATED IMPAIRMENT OF MENTAL FUNCTIONING	DECLINE IN REPUTATION OF THE COMMUNITY
LOSS OF TANGIBLES	
LOSS OF RELATIONSHIPS	

Table 1.2

Regarding overall harm, cocaine (including "crack"), methamphetamine, heroin, and alcohol were ranked as being most harmful.[29]

What I find so fascinating about these studies and dozens more like them is that they reveal there is no connection between how harmful a drug is and its legal status. A 2021 study out of the UK ranked twenty legal and illegal drugs against sixteen different harm factors. Nine criteria were harms to the users of drugs, and seven were harms to others.[30]

Table 1.2 shows the categories of harm studied:

The final results from the study were a surprise to both the researchers and the general public. It showed alcohol to be the most harmful drug overall, the most harmful to others, and the fourth most harmful to users individually.

"Many people—especially government figures—found the results challenging," remarked Dr. David Nutt. "Some criticised the findings as showing alcohol in a bad light because so many of us drink: up to 80% of the UK adult population. My riposte was that they are right—its wide use is why alcohol is the most harmful drug. And yet, it is still not legislated as such."

The reason alcohol is so frequently cited as comparable to more illicit drugs like crack, meth, and heroin is because it occupies an unfortunate "sweet spot" in world culture by being particularly dangerous while still enjoying widespread accessibility. It hurts the greatest number of people, by far.

Case in point: You don't need to be legally drunk to be cognitively affected by alcohol. Every year, drunk or "buzzed" driving is the cause of nearly 30 percent of all traffic-related deaths in the United States alone[31]—and that's likely being underreported. This means hundreds of thousands of individuals, plus their families, are being devastated by alcohol without even taking a sip. Talk about a huge ripple effect.

Despite mounting research that shows the personal and societal harm caused by alcohol, some smart people disagree.

On EP471 of his podcast, *New York Times* bestselling author and nutritionist Ben Greenfield recently explored the complexities of drinking and how it affects your health. Contrary to the AFL perspective, Ben argues that moderate consumption, around one-half to one drink per day, can actually be beneficial.[32]

He explains, "Alcohol is a toxin, but it appears that somewhere right around the range of one half to one drink per day, spread out consistently throughout the week without excess intake, is something that can be protective and beneficial."

Ben mentions the concept of hormesis, where low levels of a stressor like alcohol can apparently boost adaptation and resilience: "Alcohol causes oxidative stress, but that stress can ultimately lead to the activation of adaptive mechanisms that confer stress resilience and improve mitochondrial function."

In a nutshell: What doesn't kill you (in tiny amounts) can make you stronger.

He contrasts this moderate consumption with the risks of alcohol use disorder, noting that the harmful effects come from excessive intake, not from regular, small doses of 0.5 to 1 drink per day. "There's a big difference between having seven drinks on a Saturday night and having one drink each night of the week," he points out, emphasizing that moderation is key.

I've known Ben and been a friend for years now. I'm a big fan of his contributions, recommendations, and research in the area of health. However, on this path, we must diverge. Whether or not alcohol does create a short-term stress response that activates mitochondrial function, the net effect is you're still drinking poison.

It's doubtful most people can limit it to, as he suggests, "one-half to one drink per day." You picked up this book because you want to learn how to stop drinking, not "hack" your drinking. More to the point: Greenfield's example of moderation is still 15 to 30 drinks per month (or approximately 200 to 400 drinks per year). It seems unlikely that having 400 drinks in a year (or 4,000 in a decade) would create a positive impact on your health, no matter how much hormesis is happening.

In response to the idea of moderation with alcohol, I'm in complete agreement. The less poison you drink, the healthier you'll be.

The UK's leading biohacker, Tim Gray, says he generally doesn't drink "except once or twice a year." Gray explains that we must "pick our poison" or we won't last very long. He elaborates: "I choose to live in a city, but I filter my air and water and detoxify my body. So drinking alcohol, which is a poison, too frequently is not smart. If you want to age faster, drink. That's essentially anti-longevity. For me, I want to live longer, healthier, and happier, so I generally don't consume alcohol."

According to several thousand top performers that I've worked with over the last decade, your best bet at getting as healthy, happy, and focused as possible is to become alcohol-free. Don't shoot the messenger.

So now that you're committed to transforming your life by going alcohol-free, let's explore the different systems available to help you accomplish your goal.

FINDING A RELIABLE SYSTEM FOR QUITTING ALCOHOL

There are many different ways of quitting alcohol and there's no "one size fits all" approach; however, some systems have shown to be much more effective than others. Here are the most common ways people are offered support for quitting alcohol.

Medication-Assisted Treatment (MAT): Doctors can prescribe medications to help manage withdrawal symptoms, reduce drinking urges, or create adverse reactions to alcohol. Common medications include disulfiram (Antabuse), which makes you feel sick when you drink and naltrexone, which blocks the euphoric effects and feelings of being drunk.

These types of medications might be absolutely necessary for someone who is in imminent danger from their drinking habits. But for the average career-focused, high-achieving person reading this book, using these drugs is likely an unnecessarily drastic response. Not to mention the fact that numbing the urge to drink or the pleasure of drinking doesn't do anything to address the psychological reasons one has to drink in the first place.

Counseling / Therapy: Individuals can meet with a licensed therapist to discuss their challenges with drinking, negative thought patterns, or other issues related to their drinking. This could also be useful for couples to address the impact of drinking on the relationship.

Top performers benefit immensely from having regular access to a great therapist. I highly recommend you work with a therapist to learn more about yourself. However, many busy people may not want to spend time unpacking their entire lives just to solve a drinking habit which they don't even feel is "that bad" anyway.

Inpatient and Outpatient Rehabilitation Programs: These programs provide a controlled environment for more severe cases of alcohol dependence. Inpatient rehab includes 24-hour support and intensive care. Rehab is reserved for extreme circumstances in which a person can't stop drinking and needs a total life reset. Finally, there are 12-step programs like Alcoholics Anonymous (AA). I've reserved a special section for them because they're so popular and controversial.

WHAT ABOUT ALCOHOLICS ANONYMOUS (AA)?

AA was founded in 1935 by Bill Wilson and Dr. Bob Smith in Akron, Ohio. The organization's 12-Step program, which offers a spiritual and practical framework for overcoming addiction, has become the world's most popular method for helping people quit drinking. Through the sheer volume of results alone, you cannot discount the impact of AA. They've undoubtedly helped millions of people get clean and clear of alcohol because there's a lot they get right. They understand the incredible power of community as a catalyst for change.

I support the mission of frameworks like AA because they want people to do better, to be better, and to heal. I suspect that Alcoholics Anonymous resonates with someone who has a strong connection to their faith—or somebody who has seen others become clean through the 12 steps. Seeing others overcome alcohol up close will help you to stay strong on your own journey. There is real value in that.

However, studies suggest that 12-step programs have low long-term success rates on the whole. Dr. Lance Dodes is the former director of substance abuse treatment at Harvard's McLean Hospital and the author of the 2014 book *The Sober Truth: Debunking the Bad Science behind 12-Step Programs and the Rehab Industry*.[33]

Dodes combed through more than fifty studies and found that the success rate for Alcoholics Anonymous is between 5 and 10 percent, which he calls "one of the worst in all of medicine." AA has been so popular, so widely disseminated, that people believe it should be something that works. I'm not trying to eliminate

AA—there are undoubtedly people who have benefitted from it. I'm just saying that the numbers show it doesn't work for most people.

Recovery programs, just like every other technology, need to be updated to match the environment in which they exist. In a recent study[34] by American Addiction Centers, researchers reported:

> *National surveys suggest that of those with alcohol use disorder AUD... only about one-third attempt to quit drinking each year. Of those, only about 25% are successful at reducing their alcohol intake for more than a year... an estimated 40-60% of individuals relapsing while in recovery.*

That means if we started with one hundred people struggling with AUD, only thirty-three would attempt to quit drinking and enter treatment. Of those, only eight would be able to make it more than a year without drinking—which means 92 percent of those struggling with alcohol use disorder are not being helped by the outdated treatment methods available. That means a new, more effective approach to healing is required.

What we know from working with over two thousand clients is that understanding how your brain works and learning the neuroscience behind habit formation is the best weapon you have in your arsenal against alcohol. So, that's what we teach our community—and a study recently conducted at the University of Washington (reproduced in the appendix of this book) showed that the neuroscience-based methodology you'll learn in this book has helped clients reduce their drinking by more than 98 percent over the course of ninety days.[35] Those are the types of numbers you want to see.

For successful people, speed is a huge factor. Our clients are not interested in wasting time with programs that don't work for most people. They don't want to sit in a dusty meeting room on a Tuesday night, eating stale donuts and spilling their guts out to strangers who are chain-smoking to stop themselves from drinking. Instead, they'd much prefer to work privately with an elite team of experienced coaches, inside of a peer group with other professionals who are serious about ditching alcohol in order to get to the top of their game ASAP. If that sounds like you, then the material in this book will change your life.

DISSOLVING THE ILLUSION OF PLEASURE

Understanding why we drink is the first step toward making meaningful changes in our relationship with alcohol. The hard truth is, drinking can be a complex problem that includes social influences, psychological factors, and personal experiences that make it hard to change. You're not alone.

The approach I'm going to share with you inside this book will help you take back control of alcohol using neuroscience-based methods—without going to meetings that may leave you feeling depressed, spending thousands of dollars on rehab, or dealing with negative stigma.

Now that you know a lot more about why you drink, the next chapter will teach you step-by-step strategies for unpacking everything you've just learned and finally begin to refocus your mindset around alcohol. Over time, this mindset shift will literally rewire your brain to go from craving a drink—to enjoying abstaining from alcohol.

Ready to begin your journey to becoming alcohol-free?
Get tools, support, and free resources at
www.alcoholfreelifestyle.com/resources

KEY TAKEAWAYS

» Alcohol may feel like a friend, but it's actually a toxic influence, slowly undermining your health, progress, and success.
» You're not broken or an "alcoholic"—you're caught in a habit loop that can be rewired with the right approach.
» Drinking is deeply ingrained in human culture, making it hard to reject, but recognizing this social pressure is the first step to breaking free.

CHAPTER 1 REFLECTION POINTS

Using your favorite journal or note-taking app, write out the answers to the following prompts. These will help you bring more clarity and create simple, concrete action steps for your alcohol-free journey.

Reflection: What are the specific reasons I turn to alcohol in moments of stress or social pressure?

Question: How has my perception of alcohol as a source of comfort or connection impacted my personal or professional relationships?

Next Step: If alcohol were not an option, what healthier coping mechanisms or habits could I explore to address these triggers?

"FIFTY-THREE AND ALCOHOL-FREE: HOW I LOST SIXTY-TWO POUNDS AND CYCLED 10,000 MILES"

By Steve Aguiar
Environmental Compliance Supervisor
Elk Grove, California

WHEN COVID STARTED, I MADE a decision to stop drinking and get support doing so. What happened over the following years, I still can hardly believe. Neither can my wife, my former colleagues, and friends. They're in awe. I'm fifty-five years old. I worked for the City of Livermore in California in environmental compliance. I dealt with wastewater and stormwater regulations. I'd been doing it for twenty-seven years. Just before I got support for stopping drinking, I felt a negative vibe with my job.

I didn't like my commute on the train. I was feeling somewhat disgruntled. And I was drinking. I'm always the guy that could go big with drinking. I wasn't a one or two drink guy. I wasn't only drinking on the weekends. I was the guy who'd have two beers and a shot on the way home from work. Then I'd arrive home and have two or three more beers. That was starting to become a nightly pattern.

On one of my off Fridays, my wife returned home from her workday, realized I was drunk, and started getting teary-eyed. She said to me, "What are you doing?" I could see her concern. I could see the sadness in her eyes. It was moving for me to see her concern. When someone you care about confronts you—and not in a combative way, but with real, genuine concern because she loves you—that made me totally decide to pump the brakes on my drinking.

I didn't keep it a secret from my staff. I said, "Hey, I'm doing this alcohol-free training program and I have some times where I have to be on a Zoom call with other members. And I'm doing this. And so I just wanted to let you know." And they were supportive, even if some may have been a little skeptical.

In the first thirty or so days, I noticed I felt so much clearer in my head. I wasn't foggy. I wasn't as irritable. I was focused. And I definitely felt more positive. I just was in a better mood. I got a lot of compliments from colleagues that have known me through the years through the ups and downs of life, and they would say things like, "What are you doing? You seem so great. You have such a great positive attitude."

Before I stopped drinking, I was overweight, I had very high blood pressure, and I was on medicine for gout because I experienced gout attacks. The day I stopped drinking, March 15, 2020, I tracked my blood pressure. It was 178/111, which is really high and not good at all. On August 15, 2022—almost thirty months later—my blood pressure had dropped dramatically to 111/73. That's an incredible drop. I did not take any medicine for blood pressure. I only stopped drinking alcohol. I no longer take medication for gout. Today, I take zero pre-scription medications and am very grateful and proud of that fact.

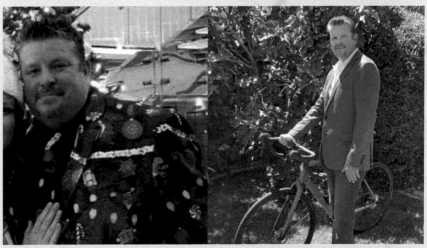

Steve lost alcohol and found a lifelong healthy habit in cycling.

My weight when I stopped drinking was 257 pounds. Today, I hover around 195 pounds. That's a 62-pound loss. I used to be a casual bike rider, cycling three miles from the train station to my office. In 2019, I cycled 500 miles. In 2020, when I stopped drinking, I cycled 5,000 miles. Then, in 2021, I doubled that distance and clocked 10,000 miles. I fell in love with cycling during my alcohol-free journey and transformed into an avid cyclist. I look and feel terrific. There are times during a long ride on the tarmac when I get an overwhelming feeling of calmness, peace, and serenity. I feel strong, confident, and alive. Cycling has given me all the things I've been seeking and which alcohol had been stripping from me.

I realize what a relief it is for my wife to see me alcohol-free. She's not worrying and can enjoy herself. It's also made me more willing to do little things for her. My mother-in-law was in a care facility, and my wife was responsible for managing all of her affairs. In the past, I'd be annoyed or put out that she was busy having to run around burdened with taking care of all the tasks associated with her mother's affairs. Quite frankly, I would simply check out, typically by having a few beers and mindlessly watching my San Francisco Giants on TV in the evening.

However, now that I am alcohol-free, I'm aware of the stress and the workload that had fallen upon her. I recognize when she's having a bad day and things are starting to overwhelm her. Now, instead of adding to this stress, I look for ways to help. I've found that just doing the little things around the house such as doing the dishes or preparing dinner make a difference. When I was drinking, I didn't care enough to take action. Now I do. Those little gestures make a big difference. I'm just a better husband.

I'm most proud of the fact that a colleague told me I inspired him to stop drinking. He came to me a few years ago and said, "I've seen what you've been doing and I've got to make changes in my own life, too. I'm going to stop drinking." I'm happy to say that person right now is coming up on four years alcohol-free himself. That's by far one of the things I'm most proud of.

I truly don't feel like I'm giving something up now. I'm gaining so much by choosing to be alcohol-free. Professionally, being alcohol-free has helped me make decisions. The clarity and the focus put me in a position to retire.

When I was drinking, I was doing the same old thing. Going to work, riding the train back and forth, not really planning for the future. I was just coexisting and believing life was happening to me. I was just getting through the day instead of planning. But now that I've been alcohol-free, I've sat down with my wife, we set the path to retire and I did it. We were proactive about it. It feels really good.

CHAPTER 2:

HOW TO REFOCUS YOUR MINDSET AROUND ALCOHOL

*"The secret of change is to focus
all your energy, not on fighting
the old, but on building the new."*

—SOCRATES

Have you ever wondered if the reason you haven't been able to reduce or quit alcohol entirely is because you're afraid to stop drinking? Your struggles with alcohol are unique, but the way those struggles make you feel isn't. In fact, thousands of my clients have expressed their very real fears over the years about what leaving alcohol behind will mean for them.

"Every obstacle is unique to each of us," offers author Ryan Holiday in his book *The Obstacle Is the Way*. "But the responses they elicit are the same: Fear. Frustration. Confusion. Helplessness. Depression. Anger. You know what you want to do but it feels like some invisible enemy has you boxed in, holding you down with pillows. You try to get somewhere, but something invariably blocks the path."[36]

Maybe you're afraid that you'll lose friends, important business opportunities, or even the potential to have a great time socially when you stop drinking. Perhaps you're afraid to deal with the internal struggle that often accompanies changing a deeply embedded habit. Many people are afraid to have difficult conversations they've been avoiding with their partners, friends or children for years of drinking. They feel like they need the alcohol to keep the pain at bay.

Flip the script: You're not losing; you're gaining. The only thing you sacrifice when you stop drinking is guaranteed mediocrity and missed connection with your loved ones. You are giving yourself and your family a gift by leaving alcohol behind. And it starts in your mind.

THE POWER OF PERCEPTION AND NEUROPLASTICITY

Even top performers who are used to being successful at most things can really struggle with quitting alcohol. I won't lie to you and promise that the process is always going to be a walk in the park—it's not. However, it's much simpler if you have proven mental frameworks for navigating the process. In order to change a deeply embedded habit around alcohol, you're going to have to learn exactly what to say when you talk to yourself.

Psychologist Shad Helmstetter said it best in his classic work *What to Say When You Talk to Yourself*: "The programming in your mind—your real 'self-talk'—is the single most powerful weapon you have to help you succeed."[37]

Shifting from a fear-based thought pattern to a positive, action-taking thought pattern can make a world of difference while you're retraining your brain to break the alcohol habit loop. For example:

Instead of thinking: *"I won't have a good time if I'm not drinking tonight."*

Say this to yourself: *"I'm looking forward to gaining a clearer mind and a healthier body tonight."*

Changing your internal language patterns can immediately alter how you perceive quitting and help you see it as an opportunity rather than a sacrifice. This isn't just because positive affirmations feel good—it's because repeatedly telling yourself something actually changes your brain through a process called neuroplasticity.

Neuroplasticity is the brain's ability to reorganize itself by forming new neural connections throughout life. It enables us to learn from and adapt to different experiences. Many people think that it's harder to learn when you're no longer a kid, but this remarkable adaptability isn't limited to childhood; it occurs at any age whenever we learn something new or modify our behavior.[38] When you repeat a task or thought patterns, the brain increases the efficiency by which these signals are sent by strengthening the connections between neurons.

If you continually tell yourself that quitting drinking will be easy while reaffirming how much you're looking forward to a clearer mind and body, these thoughts will become more dominant over time and that will indeed make the process of quitting subjectively easier[39]. Studies suggest that happier individuals, who often engage in positive thinking and affirmations, show different brain responses to emotional stimuli compared to those who are more negative.

For example, a fascinating bit of research published in the scientific journal *Social Cognitive and Affective Neuroscience* from 2016 showed that positive mental affirmations created increased activity in key regions of the brain related to self-processing and valuation that were visible via FMRI neuroimaging scans— and that participants who exhibited those increases in brain activity also showed a steep decline in sedentary behavior.[40] Essentially, what you focus on grows stronger in your neural architecture—and that can change your emotional and behavioral responses over time.

Many top performers and entrepreneurs I work with see alcohol as a necessary part of doing business—or at least use it as a social lubricant. You might have even caught yourself thinking that you need a drink to have fun and fit in.

The key to long-term success with quitting alcohol is changing the thought pattern from "I need alcohol to _____" to "I can enjoy socializing and connecting with others without alcohol."

Once you crack the code and make the switch, there's no going back. You'll begin to see social events as opportunities to build genuine connections without the crutch of alcohol, and you will legitimately have more fun as a result. I guarantee it.

Here's how you can capitalize on the amazing power of neuroplasticity to begin implementing changes immediately.

REPROGRAMMING YOUR SELF-TALK AROUND ALCOHOL

Words are powerful. If you're a religious person, you might know the phrase "In the beginning was the Word." As we speak, so we create. If every word you say and every thought you think is a brick in the palace of your intention, you must be mindful of what you're building. Let's use your tremendous creative power for good.

Destructive language patterns keep you stuck in the drinking loop. Constructive language patterns, plus direct action, will set you free.

Here's a fun exercise to try that will demonstrate how your brain works:

Roughly ten seconds from now, I want you to close your eyes and try NOT to think about a pink elephant. I repeat: Whatever you do, under absolutely no circumstances should you think about a pink elephant.

Okay, close your eyes for about five seconds.

Now they're open again.

So, what happened? I bet you thought about a pink elephant. It's impossible not to, because I already seeded your mind with the image. There's actually a scientific reason for this phenomenon called Hebb's rule.

In his 1949 book *The Organization of Behavior*,[41] Canadian neuropsychologist Dr. Donald Hebb posited what came to be known as Hebb's rule: the idea that "what fires together, wires together." This means that if two neurons are activated simultaneously, the strength of the synaptic connection between them is likely to increase. Because of Hebb's rule, we now understand how the reticular activating system (RAS) works.

The reticular activating system (RAS) is a bundle of nerves at your brainstem that filters out unnecessary information so the important stuff gets through. It plays a crucial role in regulating wakefulness and sleep-wake transitions.[42] The RAS is essentially a brain gatekeeper, constantly deciding which sensory information is important enough to process and which isn't.

When you try not to think of something, like the pink elephant, the RAS focuses on that very thing. This is because the RAS doesn't process negatives directly; it processes your focal points. So when you say "don't think about a pink elephant," your brain skips the "don't" and hears "pink elephant." Thus, the RAS zeroes in on that image even though you intended to avoid it. The reticular activating system explains why skiers who try to avoid hitting trees often steer toward and collide into them instead. When you fixate on something, you often get more of what you don't want. What you focus on focuses on you. It's the same with alcohol.

The RAS can be trained over time with mindfulness and attention practices to filter out some of your habitual thoughts, such as cravings or negative self-talk about drinking. This is why setting clear, positive intentions and using affirmative language can help reprogram your RAS, focusing your brain's attention on healthier, more constructive patterns.

If you constantly say things to yourself like:

"Don't drink."

"You better not drink again."

"We're not drinking tonight."

"Why can't you just stop drinking?"

"Not drinking is going to be so hard."

What are you focusing on more than anything else in each of these thoughts?

Drinking, of course.

Sure, you're telling yourself "not" to drink—but your brain doesn't hear the negation, it just becomes fixated on drinking. This makes you much more likely to drink.

Another quick example: How do you feel when you say the phrase "I have to..."?

Has it ever been followed by something that truly excites you?

"I have to pay my taxes."

"I have to go out to dinner with my mother-in-law."

"I have to take my kid to get a root canal."

No, thank you.

"I have to..." implies that it's hard work. It implies struggle and strain. With "have to," there is a sense of being forced or pressured. There's no out. There's ingrained resistance in the words.

You don't "have to" quit drinking. Quitting is something you choose. It's something you "get" to do.

"Trying to..." is another famous trap, keeping you stuck in a wishy-washy commitment instead of holding a clear, strong intention. When you say "try," it implies the possibility of failure for reasons outside of your control. Yet your habits—even your deeply embedded ones—are 100 percent within your control.

As Jedi Master Yoda famously said in the 1980 film *The Empire Strikes Back*: "Do or do not, there is no try."

Now, let's flip the switch. Imagine how you'd feel if you simply changed the language pattern from "have to..." or "trying to..." to "I choose to..." or "I get to..." or even "I'm so fortunate/grateful/ happy that..."

For instance...

Imagine you're attending a party and you know everyone is going to be drinking. Instead of focusing on the fact that you "can't" have alcohol, redirect your thoughts to what you're choosing to enjoy—and why.

Before you get to the party, you might say to yourself something like, "I'm going to have a great time with friends, eat delicious food, and enjoy some mocktails because I want to feel fresh in the morning." This shift focuses your mindset on the positive aspects of an alcohol-free night by opening up new possibilities for enjoyment without alcohol. And it attaches a benefit-driven reason to what you're doing.

You may even want to literally rehearse the lines out loud before getting to the event: "I'll take a club soda with lime, thank you very much." Say it ten times in the mirror. Get used to the feeling of the words in your mouth. Instead of saying, "I'm really trying to quit drinking," say, "I love my daily soda water and lime because it makes me feel healthy and hydrated." Simple, affirmative, and benefit-driven.

Now that you understand more about how your self-talk around alcohol affects your consumption patterns, let's look a little closer at how cues, routines and rewards become the building blocks of our most deeply ingrained habits.

UNDERSTANDING CUES, ROUTINES, AND REWARDS

Habit change is a science, but it doesn't happen overnight. In his bestselling book *Atomic Habits*, author James Clear describes the process of slow change as a gradual shift, not an instantaneous improvement[43]:

> As you continue to layer small changes on top of one another, the scales of life start to move. Each improvement is like adding a grain of sand to the positive side of the scale, slowly tilting things in your favor. Eventually, if you stick with it, you hit a tipping point.

This is how small changes create massive wins over time.

As we discussed in Chapter 1, habits are formed through a cycle known as the habit loop, which consists of three components: the cue, the routine, and the reward. This cycle plays a pivotal role in the development of alcohol habits. By understanding how it works, you can learn to control it for your benefit. Let's dig in:

The cue: this is the trigger that initiates the habit. Cues are the reasons why you want to pick up a drink in the first place. A cue can be external or internal.

External cues are situational and environmental triggers. Attending social events where alcohol is flowing freely, seeing an advertisement for alcohol on TV, or being offered a drink by a friend are all examples of powerful external cues. Even the *pfft* sound of opening a can of beer or the pop of a wine cork can act as an external cue. External cues are so powerful because they are linked to specific contexts where drinking is a normalized behavior.[44]

External cues sound like: *"Every time I do, see or hear [INSERT CUE], it makes me want to drink."*

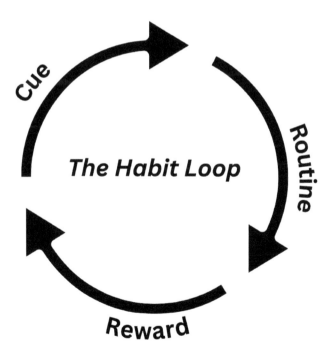

The habit loop as originally described by Charles Duhigg.

Internal cues involve your emotional and psychological states. Feeling negative emotions like anxiety, sadness, stress, loneliness, or boredom can all be strong internal cues to pick up a drink. Internal cues are deeply personal and can be harder to identify because they involve introspection and self-awareness. Recognizing these cues is crucial for addressing the root causes of habitual drinking.

Internal cues sound like: "*Every time I feel or experience [INSERT CUE], it makes me want to drink.*"

The routine: the behavior itself—in this case, consuming alcohol.

When faced with the cue (an environment or feeling), you automatically begin to follow the routine (drinking) to address the cue. Your brain follows a simple logic program of "If X, then Y." You might as well call the program "RunDrinking.exe."

This routine becomes more automatic over time, requiring less conscious thought. The routine of drinking can become ingrained, making it a default response to certain cues. For instance, if someone routinely drinks a glass of wine every evening to unwind after a stressful day, this behavior becomes an automatic response to the cue of evening relaxation time. You might run the following program five days a week: When [I'm stressed after a long day of work], then I [pour myself a gigantic glass of red wine].

This repeated programming makes it more difficult to break your habit because the brain has formed strong neural connections that reinforce the behavior and actually rewards the loop a la Hebb's rule.[45]

Reward: the positive reinforcement that follows the routine.

Alcohol provides a temporary sense of pleasure, relaxation, or escape from negative emotions. The temporary stress relief is a reward your brain craves, so it strengthens the association between the cue and the routine. Over time, the brain starts to anticipate the reward whenever the cue is present, making the habit more ingrained.[46]

Adding to the logic above:

When [I'm stressed after a long day of work], then I [pour myself a gigantic glass of red wine] = [I feel more relaxed]

The upside of drinking alcohol is that the reward is often immediate, providing quick relief from stress or anxiety. About five minutes into a glass of whiskey, you will begin to forget your problems—and that's quite encouraging.

The downside is that while the immediate reward may be pleasurable, the long-term consequences of habitual drinking can be severe. You're not actually solving any of the problems you're using alcohol to run away from by drinking. But you already knew that.

Homer Simpson from the TV series *The Simpsons* said it best: "Beer. Now there's a temporary solution."

Now that you understand how cues, routines and rewards come together to form a habit loop with alcohol, you can reverse engineer the process. It's time to take an active approach and consciously create new, positive habits in your life.

PRACTICAL EXAMPLES OF STAYING ALCOHOL-FREE IN EVERYDAY SCENARIOS

Transformation is an inside job. Even though you've decided not to drink, alcohol will still be everywhere. That's one reason this journey can be so challenging for my clients. By quitting drinking, you're learning to change your own mindset and internal programming while the environment around you continues to exist unchanged.

To accomplish your goal, you'll need to mentally prepare for the most common situations you're likely to encounter. If you plan how you'll handle the temptation to drink in advance, you'll be more self-aware and confident about your decision not to drink, no matter what environment you find yourself in.

DEALING WITH WORK AND
LIFE STRESS WITHOUT ALCOHOL

My clients are executives, professionals, and entrepreneurs who work in high-pressure, demanding careers. For these types of top performers, alcohol is often used as a release valve to unwind after a stressful day. I don't blame them for wanting to relax. When you're responsible for a lot at work, the challenges and to-do lists are endless.

The question is: How do you unwind from a predictably stressful day without alcohol at the center? The first step is becoming aware of the cues that are leading you to drink.

Eliminate External Cues in Your Environment

When you walk in your kitchen, is the first thing you see a gigantic wine bottle ready to be poured? Does your home have a mini-bar that rivals the penthouse suite of a luxury hotel? Are the glass bottles in your weekly recycling bin made up of mostly alcohol bottles? If so, it's time for a home detox.

Clear out all the alcohol in your home. Just get rid of it. If you're sick about how much money you're "wasting," take comfort in the fact the money has already been spent. Now, you're just sparing yourself the health consequences. Next, clear out any reminders of alcohol in your house. Old bottles, wine glasses, boxes. Trash them. Eliminate all potential triggers. Stock your house with a variety of nonalcoholic beverages you enjoy. Remind yourself, "I love how energized and clearheaded I feel without alcohol." Experiment with making your own mocktails or trying new herbal teas to find satisfying alternatives to alcohol.

Observe Internal Cues In Your Mind

What types of thought patterns lead you to picking up a drink after work? For most people, the main culprits are stress, overwhelm and fatigue. Take a moment to observe the things you think or say to yourself before having a drink at home. For instance, if you catch yourself saying something like:

>> "I can't wait until I get home so that I can have a big glass of Malbec."
>> "Today was really rough. Just a little something to take the edge off."
>> "I'm so stressed. I deserve this beer."

STOP. Recognize these as cues to drink. Take a brief pause, not to criticize yourself, but to become curious about your own internal cues. Get excited that you were able to recognize a cue before it turned into a routine. By recognizing these thought patterns before acting on them, you're shining a bright light on triggers that were previously subconscious.

Next, begin to unravel your habit by asking yourself questions to get to the root of your urge to drink. Here are a few examples of questions you can ask yourself that will dig into your own motivations for drinking. Feel free to make your own variations:

>> "Do I really even want to drink?"
>> "Why do I want to drink right now?"
>> "What feelings am I trying to escape with alcohol?"
>> "How will alcohol make my situation / problem worse?"
>> "Am I being honest with myself about my relationship with alcohol?"
>> "How have I seen this pattern / habit with alcohol played out in the past?"
>> "How does drinking make me feel about myself?"

Once you've become aware of the primary cues that trigger you to drink when you're stressed, you can actively install a new routine in place of drinking.

Installing Alcohol-Free Routines

Anything that appeals to you can replace the routine of drinking alcohol. The good thing about quitting is that it'll give you more time, money and energy back to reinvest into something new.

If you primarily use alcohol as a way to calm your nerves, try replacing it with a habit to help you calm down and emotionally regulate. For example:

» Meditation or a mindfulness routine
» Prayer
» Yoga
» Deep breathing exercises
» Take a relaxing bath or get a massage

If you drink primarily to forget about the stress of the day, consider a creative habit to get you into a flow state:

» Journaling or writing
» Drawing, painting or other crafts
» Cooking or baking a new recipe
» Learning a new skill, instrument or hobby
» Reading a book

If you use alcohol as a mood booster, try something more active such as:

» Go for a walk or run
» Lift weights or take a fitness class
» Train a martial art like Brazilian Jiu Jitsu
» Play outside with your dog or kids

Your new habit loop could look like this:

When [I'm stressed after a long day of work], then I [meditate for twenty minutes] = [I feel more relaxed and centered]

That's a huge win. And the best part is, you won't get cancer from meditation.

If you're intrigued, but don't know where to start, don't worry. It doesn't matter if you know anything about meditation, have never taken a music lesson in your life or you've not stepped inside a gym for a while. Now that you're not drinking, you can get into the groove. There are YouTube videos, classes and communities for anything you could possibly want to learn. Take this opportunity to level up your skills outside of work and develop new areas of yourself.

When you are feeling stressed from the day, instead of using alcohol to take the edge off, intentionally steer your focus into one of these new routines. These activities offer the same emotional state changes you're looking for from alcohol (feeling more calm, flowing, happy, etc.) without all the toxic downstream effects. Sure, alcohol's effects might come on a bit faster than some of the routines listed above, but you have to keep drinking to ride the wave.

If you replace drinking every evening after work with a twenty-minute workout, you'll begin to release endorphins that will make you feel less stressed almost immediately—and the effects are long-lasting. Plus, you'll have the added benefit of doing something extremely healthy for your body. The long-term positive effects these new, positive routines have on your life quickly outweigh the temporary reward of a happy buzz that alcohol provides.

Remain aware of the cues that trigger the urge to drink and install better habits. That sounds simple enough. But what about when you're out with friends or family and they're encouraging you to drink?

ATTENDING A PARTY OR SOCIAL EVENT WITHOUT ALCOHOL

It can be jarring to experience social events without alcohol because it's so normalized in our culture. If friends or family are drinking, it feels comfortable to join in. I invite you to use this opportunity to observe how you interact with others alcohol-free—and I encourage you to notice how you're still able to have fun without being drunk.

Before attending the event, review in your mind your intention to be alcohol-free and use positive language to affirm exactly why you won't be drinking.

"I'm looking forward to being completely clear tonight so that I can get a jump on my priorities tomorrow."

If you're going to a gathering where everyone is bringing some sort of food or beverage, bring your favorite nonalcoholic drinks. Perhaps a refreshing kombucha, sparkling water or tea? All restaurants and bars will have some sort of nonalcoholic beverage selection. When you're not sure, just order a club soda with lime. For your reference, there's a list of twenty-two refreshing alcohol-free drinks you can make at home in Appendix A of this book.

I personally like the Colorado-based alcohol-free drinks brand Grüvi. Co-founders and brother-and-sister duo Niki and Anika Sawni have created a collection of very good alcohol-free craft beers and wines. Full disclosure: I'm an investor.

Practice the line to yourself so that your response to "what would you like to drink?" is automatic.

"Club soda with lime, thank you."

BEWARE OF SMILING ASSASSINS

In the AFL community, we have a special name for people who try to get us to drink.

We call them Smiling Assassins. These assassins are smiling as they hand you a drink that's slowly killing you. It could be your mother, your father, your best friend, your colleagues or your boss.

Hey, would you like a drink?

Can I get you a drink?

Let's go out for drinks!

How about a beer?

They're all grinning as they're encouraging you to guzzle attractively packaged poison. It's all part of the indoctrination. Don't take the bait.

Envision what your friends or family might say when they realize you're not drinking tonight. Are you worried about their judgement? If so, take a deep breath and realize that nobody cares.

Although you might be worried about others judging you for not drinking, the honest-to-God truth is that nobody cares. Most people are completely absorbed in their own life and will not even notice the changes you're making in yours. There may be little or no reaction to your decision to go alcohol-free—in which case, any anxiety about what others might think was a complete waste of energy.

Even if they say something like:

"Come on, can't you just have one?"

"Wow, you're no fun."

"I'm not taking no for an answer."

"It's rude not to drink when others are drinking."

"You're going to make me be the only one drinking?"

"Studies have shown alcohol is good for _____."

"One won't kill ya!"

"What's wrong, can't handle your alcohol?"

Who cares? Don't let it bother you.

Simply respond with something that makes your intentions clear. You can even use a little humor to lighten the mood:

"I'm not drinking tonight. I've had enough beer to last a lifetime, don't you think?"

"I'm working on getting healthier right now. I'm cutting alcohol for a bit to see if I can get abs."

You can also simply say: *"No thanks, I'm good for now."*

Remember one thing: When others try to goad you into drinking, it's because they don't want to be the only one poisoning themselves in order to have "fun." It's not about you, it's about them. Deep down in our hearts, humans know instinctively that alcohol is poison because of how bad hangovers feel. By taking a break from alcohol, you're simply listening to the voice that was already there.

Now that you're at an event alcohol-free, have fun. Join into conversations, listen to others, play games, listen to music, etc. As the event continues, you'll notice that nobody will ask you about why you're not drinking. Nobody cares.

NAVIGATING PROFESSIONAL SITUATIONS WITHOUT ALCOHOL

With all the top performers, entrepreneurs and executives I've coached, their objective is always to do the absolute best work they can. It's this relentless drive to become better that's gotten them to where they are in life—and many are still looking to find an edge in their fifties, sixties, and beyond.

If you are in a professional situation and you are the only person who isn't drinking, you have a measurable competitive advantage in your ability to reason and recall information against everybody else in the room. For this reason alone, quitting alcohol is a secret weapon to spring past your peers and upgrade your professional status.

Preparing for Professional Events

Are you planning to go to a dinner, meeting or professional outing that will likely include booze? Are you concerned that you'll be tempted to drink (like always)?

First: remember that you do not need alcohol to be personable or charismatic. You don't need to drink to get others to like you, get a promotion or to close a deal. If you do find one of those to be true, you should begin looking for another job.

If you know that not drinking at the event is going to be very challenging, set clear boundaries for yourself and prepare your mind in advance by deciding on nonalcoholic drinks. Affirm to yourself, "I choose to stay sharp and focused by drinking club soda with lime tonight."

Prepare yourself by reviewing your intentions for the event. Ask yourself "what's my purpose at this event?"

- » Are you there to close a deal?
- » Are you there to network?
- » Are you there to hire or recruit?
- » Are you there to promote?

Whatever the intention is, put all your focus on that. If you have a clear purpose for why you are attending an event, it will help you stay more present during the process—and you're much more likely to get what you want out of the interactions.

The biggest piece of advice I can give you to succeed in social or professional situations is to display a fun and carefree attitude toward being alcohol-free. Have confidence and conviction about your decision to change your life for the better. How you share with others that you're not drinking is far more important than whatever words come out of your mouth. There's no need to be so serious about it—you're not announcing a death sentence. Choosing not to drink is a very good decision and pretty much everybody knows it. Be confident in your decision and others will respect it.

Studies have shown that persuading and influencing people is rarely about what you say and mostly about how you say it. In fact, influencing others comes down to 55 percent visual cues, 38 percent tone, and only 7 percent words.[47]

Whenever I want to communicate a calm feeling of confidence, I think of George Clooney's cheeky, confident grin. If you haven't watched Ocean's 11, you're missing out. Next time you're in a social setting, put on your best George Clooney smile and make a joke about the fact that you're not drinking. If someone mocks you (which rarely happens), say, "Yeah, I'm going to get drunk on this water tonight. I am going to swing from the rafters. Look out, I am going to go crazy on this soda water tonight."

(I don't condone megastars like George Clooney, Ryan Reynolds, and Dwayne "The Rock" Johnson pushing their brands of attractively packaged poison—but I can take notes from their confident swagger.)

When people see that you're confident about your decision, they will stop encouraging you to drink. If people still persist—"Come on, just have one!"—grin and confidently reply, "No, I'm good, thank you."

WHAT HAPPENS IF YOU SLIP?

It's possible that you will read this book, follow all the steps and suggestions inside for quitting alcohol, and still end up having a drink at some point down the road. Old habits die hard. Please realize that changing your relationship with alcohol is not a "zero sum" game. You get credit for each day you're not drinking.

Here's why you don't need to be perfect: for every day that you're not drinking, you're actually saving your body from the negative health impact of all the drinks you would have likely had. It adds up. So if you slip and have a drink, don't spend time criticizing yourself. One drink doesn't negate or undo the positive health benefits of the twenty alcohol-free days before it. Just remain aware so that one night doesn't turn into a second night, and then every night again. Recognize that you're in the process of a habit change process and get right back to it the next day. Do not mourn your mistakes.

Think about extending your alcohol-free streak one day at a time. Imagine your new lifestyle is a video game where you're collecting points for each day you're alcohol-free. That will take the pressure off. The longer you can keep the streak going, the more points you rack up. A full month of not drinking is saving the negative health impact of dozens of drinks on your body. Imagine the stress you're saving your kidneys, liver, immune system, heart, brain...and wallet.

One of the best ways to get back on track after you have a drink is to talk to somebody who genuinely wants to see you succeed. An encouraging word, a story of mutual struggle or a simple hug is often all we need to remember the world isn't over and get back on the horse. The old proverb says "if you want to go fast, go alone. If you want to go far, go together." Stop trying to do everything alone. Share your goals with family, friends or a community as a way of accountability and ask for support in becoming alcohol-free. When life seems especially hard, good relationships will always get you through.

"Relationships are all there is," says leadership and networking expert Keith Ferrazzi in his breakthrough book *Never Eat Alone*. "Everything in the universe only exists because it is in relationship to everything else. Nothing exists in isolation. We have to stop pretending we are individuals that can go it alone."[48]

If you're having trouble quitting drinking, know that you're not alone. Once you share your goal to quit drinking with others, even the fact that others know will encourage you to stay on track because now others are invested. Sharing with others may also encourage them to try the alcohol-free lifestyle as well, which will create even more reinforcement and accountability within your social group. Surround yourself with people who want to succeed and your success is much more likely.

BECOME AN ALCOHOL-FREE SUPERHERO

One simple psychological hack you can employ to speed up the process of change is creating a new identity (or alter ego) around the version of yourself who doesn't drink. Peak performance coach Todd Herman explains the concept brilliantly in his book *The Alter Ego Effect*:

> *An Alter Ego is simply a trusted friend inside of you. It's a phenomenal creative imagination technique that's been used for centuries by some of history's most successful people. It's a way to use other sides of you that already exist to increase your performance and happiness. You don't have to create something false—there's nothing fake about it. You're just uncovering the hero already inside yourself by leveraging an Alter Ego to bring it out.*[49]

I had so much more fun doing new things alcohol-free. I suppose this was due to the fact that I began to see myself as a different person. It was an alter ego of the old James. And this version had much more energy available for me to do new and interesting activities because my body and brain weren't busy constantly cleaning up the damage alcohol had done. It was like a hardware and software upgrade at the same time.

HOW TO CREATE YOUR ALTER EGO

1. **Define Your Purpose:** Identify what you want to achieve with your alter ego. Consider areas where you want to improve, like confidence or assertiveness.

2. **Select Your Superpowers:** Determine the traits you want your alter ego to embody (e.g., fearless, charismatic, resilient). List adjectives that describe how you want to show up in challenging situations.

3. **Craft a Name:** Choose a name that resonates with the qualities of your alter ego. It could be a combination of names, a title (like "Commander"), or even an animal name. Consider a name that has emotional resonance for you to strengthen your connection to it.

4. **Create an Origin Story:** Develop a backstory for your alter ego that explains its strengths and motivations. Use this story to connect emotionally and provide context for your alter ego's traits.

5. **Visualize the Transformation:** Picture how you would act, think, and feel as your alter ego in various situations. How would your body language change? What thoughts would you have? Visualize different social scenarios to reinforce this identity.

6. **Practice Activation:** Create rituals or use physical totems (like specific clothing or objects) to activate your alter ego before entering challenging situations. This helps reinforce the mindset and characteristics associated with your alter ego.

7. **Experiment and Adapt:** Use your alter ego in real-life situations to see how it influences your performance. Be open to refining your alter ego as you grow and learn more about yourself.

8. **Maintain a Lighthearted Approach:** Keep the process fun and enjoyable to avoid feeling trapped or forced. Use your alter ego as a tool for exploration and creativity in your alcohol-free journey.

IT'S TIME TO TAKE YOUR
POWER BACK FROM ALCOHOL

Refocusing your mindset around alcohol is a powerful step toward embracing an alcohol-free lifestyle. By changing your perception, using positive, benefit-driven language, and understanding the science of habit formation, you can successfully navigate the journey to being completely alcohol-free. Use these tools and you'll find that quitting alcohol is not an act of deprivation—but a gift to yourself.

Now that you have a clearer picture of exactly why you drink and how to change your mindset around alcohol, we'll be able to get into the good stuff. In Part II of this book, we will explore how the Alcohol-Free Lifestyle can expand and transform the four pillars of your life: health, wealth, relationships, and happiness.

We'll dig deep and discuss the uncomfortable truth about how alcohol negatively impacts these areas. Then I'll show you exactly what your life will look like when you finally give it up for good.

Get excited. You're on your way to a happier, healthier, and wealthier life.

Ready to begin your journey to becoming alcohol-free?
Get tools, support, and free resources at
www.alcoholfreelifestyle.com/resources

KEY TAKEAWAYS

» The way you talk to yourself matters—saying "I choose to be alcohol-free" makes quitting feel empowering instead of restrictive.
» Focusing on not drinking keeps alcohol on your mind—shift your focus to positive alternatives like feeling energized and enjoying new experiences.
» Breaking the habit of drinking takes time, but by creating new routines, you can rewire your brain and build healthier patterns.

CHAPTER 2 REFLECTION POINTS

Write out the answers to the following prompts in your favorite journal to create simple, concrete action steps for your alcohol-free journey.

Reflection: What beliefs about alcohol have I inherited from family, friends, or society, and how have they shaped my behavior?

Question: How does my current relationship with alcohol align with the vision I have for my best self?

Next Step: What is one empowering thought I can adopt today to begin changing my mindset about alcohol?

"HEALING MY TRAUMA AND EMBRACING LIMITLESS POSSIBILITIES WITHOUT ALCOHOL"

By Karen Grundhofer
Technology Consultant and Philanthropist
Newport Beach, California

M Y JOURNEY TO BECOME ALCOHOL-FREE began as a way to cope with the anxiety and pain from extremely traumatic experiences, particularly being a gunshot victim in a college shooting. Despite my best efforts, including two years of sobriety through Alcoholics Anonymous (AA), I never found true freedom from alcohol.

I felt like I was white-knuckling it, always longing for a drink. I couldn't understand why I was still so unhappy. I identified as a survivor, but being labeled as an "alcoholic" never sat right with me. I wanted alcohol out of my life, but AA wasn't the answer I needed.

That changed when I found the support group, Alcohol-Free Lifestyle. Finally, I had the tools and understanding I needed to quit drinking for good. Now, celebrating being alcohol-free since 2022, I can honestly say these past years have been the best of my life.

I used alcohol to soothe my anxiety and pain. It became my best friend, but deep down, I knew it was only holding me back. I was living in a constant state of fight or flight, never fully dealing with the trauma that haunted me. Alcohol was my way of surviving, not living.

Free from the grip of alcohol, I feel a profound sense of purpose and joy. My story is one of resilience, growth, and the power of finding the right support system to overcome life's most difficult challenges. Today, I am not just a survivor; I am thriving and committed to helping others find their own paths to freedom.

I went from feeling trapped and powerless to truly free and in control of my life. It's like I've been given a second chance at living, and I'm not looking back. I'm excited about what the future holds. Now that I'm in this place of growth, I want to stay here forever. The possibilities are limitless.

PART II:

THE CASE
FOR GOING
ALCOHOL-FREE

CHAPTER 3:

HEALING THE EFFECTS OF ALCOHOL ON YOUR BRAIN AND BODY

"Whisky is a good thing in its place. There is nothing like it for preserving a man when he is dead. If you want to keep a dead man, put him in whisky; if you want to kill a live man, put whisky in him."

—THOMAS GUTHRIE

I MET FORMER NFL GREAT TERRELL Owens, popularly known by his initials, T.O., in 2010. T.O. played in the NFL for sixteen seasons, was a six-time Pro-Bowl selection and five-time first-team All-Pro, he holds or shares several NFL records, and was inducted into the Pro Football Hall of Fame in 2018.

When I met T.O., I was interviewing him for *SportsCenter* during his final NFL season. Later, I bumped into him at various industry parties, including the ESPY Awards and Golden Globes in Los Angeles and the Sundance Film Festival in Salt Lake City. At those late-night industry parties, I would always notice that he wasn't drinking alcohol.

When I asked him about his drinking habits, he told me, "I don't drink much at all, very seldom… I didn't really drink much during my playing days, none during the season and I've really kept that regimen going."

"It's a choice," he went on to say. "Being an athlete, you know what's good for your body and what's not, and I knew that alcohol wasn't going to bode well for me if I was going to be successful."

If you were a pro athlete performing at the top of your game, like T.O., you'd probably be willing to go the extra mile to give yourself every possible competitive advantage. You'd take every action to keep yourself in a state of optimum health, energy, and performance. It's not so different in the game of business.

I've noticed something interesting in many of the people I've met and worked with over the years: Entrepreneurs and high performers are very health-conscious people. They live a healthy lifestyle, devoting time, energy, and money to wellness and personal development. Yet many never stop to question the role that alcohol plays in negating that healthy lifestyle.

Eating well, exercising, and meditating while drinking regularly is like trying to move forward with one foot on the gas and one foot on the brake. You waste a lot of energy, and you don't get very far. The answer is not to accelerate even harder—it's to take your foot off the brake. Alcohol is the brake that is stalling your progress, and quitting it is one of the best things you can do for your health.

Especially when it comes to your brain.

HOW ALCOHOL AFFECTS YOUR BRAIN HEALTH

In 2019, I was a guest on my friend Max Lugavere's top health podcast, *Genius Life*, in which we talked about the health and social consequences of alcohol consumption. Max is a leading voice in cognitive health and the author of the *New York Times* best seller *Genius Foods*, in addition to *The Genius Life and Genius Kitchen*.

Despite being well-researched, it's the firsthand experience of his mother's battle with cognitive decline that has made him really understand what's at stake when we drink. "Seeing my mom's health decline made me realize how crucial it is to take care of our brains, and alcohol is one of those things that can really undermine that effort," he shared.[50]

Drinking alcohol is essentially micro-dosing poison—and your body knows it. In fact, alcohol activates microglial cells, the cells in your brain responsible for defending your central nervous system. When overactivated in the presence of alcohol, microglial cells can harm neurons instead of protecting them. When you combine this neural damage with the inflammatory response in your brain over time, cognitive decline is likely. In this way, alcohol encourages and aggravates Alzheimer's and other forms of dementia.[51]

Long-term drinking habits can cause lasting damage to brain structures, particularly the hippocampus, which is responsible for forming new memories. Studies have shown that even if you're only drinking a moderate amount, alcohol can still cause parts of it to shrink.[52] As a result, regular alcohol consumers often experience difficulties with memory recall, decision-making, and problem-solving—skills that are vital for professional success.

One of the reasons alcohol is so damaging is because it passes right through the blood-brain barrier and begins disrupting the chemicals called neurotransmitters almost instantly. This interference can lead to some pretty noticeable changes in how you think and act. It's like alcohol flips a few switches in your brain, and suddenly things aren't working as smoothly as they usually do.

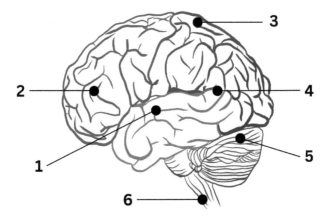

Many different regions of the brain are affected by even mild alcohol consumption. Below is a list detailing the impact of alcohol on six key areas.
1. Hippocampus: learning and memory is processed here. Drinkers can have a hard time with recall and absorbing new information.
2. Frontal lobe: alcohol can affect this area, which infl uences emotions and mood. Fluctuations can lead to anxiety and depression.
3. Cerebral cortex: Decision-making and critical thinking start here. Alcohol can impact your ability to think on your feet and make important decisions.
4. Hypothalamus and pituitary gland: alcohol can disrupt the autonomic brain functions and hormones released by these regions. Sleep patterns can be severely affected.
5. Cerebellum: the area regulates bodily coordination. Drinkers can be more clumsy even when not drinking, leading to accidents and injury.
6. Medulla: this area controls vital functions in the heart and lungs. Drinkers can have slower respiratory and heart rates, leading to problems.

DRINKING HIJACKS DOPAMINE AND OTHER VITAL NEUROTRANSMITTERS:

"My relationship with alcohol has snowballed and is getting worse," said one of our *Project 90* members. "I drink beer every night to escape reality. It's killing me—my mind, my memory, and my body." The truth is, they are absolutely right about the deleterious effects of drinking on their mind.

Here's a breakdown of how alcohol affects your neurotransmitters:

Dopamine: Dopamine is basically your brain's feel-good chemical because it exists to give you pleasure. Initially, drinking boosts your dopamine levels, which is why you get that happy or euphoric feeling. However, there's no free lunch. As you continue to drink, alcohol decreases your natural dopamine production. Now, you have to drink more and more to feel good.

This cycle can lead the brain to associate alcohol consumption with increased dopamine, forming an addictive habit loop.[53] Over time, this loop can only lead straight to hell in the form of issues like depression, reduced motivation, and an overall decline in cognitive focus.[54]

Yes, drinking can make you feel more inspired or creative for a short time. It can temporarily alleviate some of your worries. But if you're in an entrepreneurial or creative career, you don't need inspiration. Your craft relies on sustained discipline and continuous learning to produce your best work. You can't have either of those while you're on the dopamine roller coaster.

GABA (gamma-aminobutyric acid): Alcohol enhances the effects of GABA, a neurotransmitter responsible for slowing down brain activity. Changes in GABA levels are the reason for slurred speech, impaired motor skills, and delayed reaction times.[55]

If you're a top performer, you'll find yourself in many meetings where sharp thinking and clear communication are critical. And if you've ever taken a morning meeting after having a few drinks the night before, you know that your brain feels anything but sharp. This can lead to missed opportunities to make a strong impression or close a crucial deal.

(I know, because many clients have shared with me the pain of losing a deal when they were not mentally sharp after a night of drinking.)

GABA's inhibitory effects slow down your brain's processing power. This is why alcohol is classified as a depressant—not because it literally makes you "depressed," but because it puts the brakes on your brain's activity. The scary part is that these effects can be cumulative and long-term.

Glutamate: Alcohol interferes with the activity of glutamate, an essential neurotransmitter for cognitive processes like learning new information and retaining memories.[56] Glutamate is also important for something called synaptic plasticity. This is essentially your brain's way of staying flexible, which allows you to learn and remember more effectively.

Professionals need to stay sharp in order to remain competitive. That means constantly learning new information. Regular alcohol consumption slows your ability to absorb and retain new material, which can directly affect your performance at work. The last thing you want is to miss an important opportunity because you were too slow, groggy, or forgetful to take advantage of it.

Outside of the negative cognitive effects of alcohol, the setbacks can trickle down to your career in many ugly ways, significantly diminishing your ability to level up.

HOW ALCOHOL IMPACTS YOUR COGNITIVE PERFORMANCE AT WORK

Consider the case of a senior executive who is struggling to remember crucial details during board meetings because his brain is consistently foggy from the night before. At least three times a week, he goes out with clients, friends, or other executives and has two to three drinks. His focus is always scattered, and he can't create enough energy to really get his points across. His body and mind are always exhausted.

Habitual drinking is the toll that keeps on taking. Once he drops the booze, life and work will gradually get better.

Here are some of the most common ways alcohol negatively impacts your performance at work:

1. Missed Deadlines and Opportunities

Drinking often leads to procrastination, which can result in you missing deadlines and opportunities.

Imagine that you're a sales manager who routinely drinks on weeknights. Each morning, you struggle to get out of bed and feel groggy. One morning, tragedy strikes: you oversleep and miss an important meeting with a potential client for your company to sign. How do you think your company is going to react? Do you think the client will want to do business with you?

Alcohol can tend to make you drag your feet as well. When it's in your system, you may find yourself slower to respond to messages. Before you know it, you're buried under a mountain of tasks and emails. Of course, this can crank up your stress levels and make you want to drink even more to cope. It's a tough cycle that can really get in the way of your success at work.

2. Decreased Work Quality

Chronic drinking leads to fatigue and brain fog, reducing the overall quality of work you produce. You may find you lose your spark of inspiration under the heavy weight of alcohol.

Imagine an advertising executive with decades of experience who is renowned for her innovative marketing campaigns. She starts drinking wine every night after work because she believes it will help her unwind and think creatively. Over time, the opposite begins to happen. Her creativity wanes and her ideas become more repetitive. Her campaigns stop hitting hard.

The difference between the type of work she is able to create when she's drinking every night compared with what she'll be capable of once she quits is night and day. There's no question. She'll be able to think of new ideas more easily and create campaigns that actually make a difference for her company again. Instead of worrying about keeping her job, now she's getting a promotion. It's a snowball effect.

3. Poor Decision-Making

Your career is the sum total of the decisions you make. Making decisions requires you to think about many variables to choose one option above all others. Alcohol makes you effectively stupid because it impairs your judgment and critical thinking.

You might be thinking, *I can handle my alcohol. I've been drinking for years while still continuing to get promoted and praised for my work.* Be careful: this line of thinking is a top performer's trap. Just because you can perform well with alcohol in your life doesn't mean you can't perform much better without it. It's a handicap, no matter how you slice it.

TEN PROVEN PRACTICES TO HEAL YOUR BRAIN AND BODY FROM THE DAMAGING EFFECTS OF ALCOHOL

Many of the positive benefits of quitting or reducing alcohol can be felt immediately and they compound over time. That's the type of compound interest you want. Below are a few strategies you can use to begin feeling more clarity and focus on the road to success in your new alcohol-free lifestyle. You don't need to implement all of these at once or be dogmatic about them. It's not about going to extremes.

Instead, try introducing new routines into your life where they fit, reclaiming the time and energy you get from leaving the alcohol behind.

Stress is one of the biggest triggers that will tempt you to reach for a drink. It's important to be aware of this so that you are prepared to deal with stressors when they arise and have healthier alternatives to turn to.

When you're stressed after a rough day at work or you've had a fight with your partner, you're probably going to want a drink. Or, you're going to think you want a drink.

But here's the truth: You don't really want a drink. What you really want is relief from the stress that you're feeling—and you can do that without a drink. In this chapter, I outline simple but effective ways to deal with stress in a constructive way. There's nothing complicated or difficult here. We're going back to basics as we train ourselves to turn to healthier ways of coping.

1. TAPPING INTO A DAILY GRATITUDE PRACTICE

Gratitude is both a natural by-product of living alcohol-free and a conscious practice that can support an alcohol-free lifestyle. It's one of the most rewarding morning rituals I've encountered and something I make a priority of incorporating into my morning routine.

A 2003 study found that counting your blessings in a daily journal increases your ability to adapt to change, reduces physical pain, and is correlated with better sleep.[57] Another study done by Rollin McCraty demonstrated that cultivating appreciation led to a 23 percent decrease in cortisol[58] (a hormone related to stress), and 80 percent of participants experienced an increase in heart rate variability, a key indicator of health. Add this happiness hack to your walk outside and ponder two or three things you're feeling grateful for each day.

I suggest keeping a journal and writing down a list of ten things you're grateful for, big or small. You'll find that where your attention goes, energy flows. Where once you saw problems, you'll begin to see opportunities.

2. DEVELOPING A DAILY MOVEMENT PRACTICE

The word *emotion* stands for "energy in motion"—that is to say, the emotions you experience are literally energy flowing through.[59] Sometimes, the best way to clear a negative emotion is literally to work it out of your system. Move it through your body. Sweat it out through your pores. It really works.

When you exercise, it changes your state because your mind is distracted from your problems as you're focused on the present. You can use physical activity to drown out the negative voice in your head with a flood of endorphins—another type of neurotransmitter that's released in response to exercise. Not only does the high of exercise last longer than that of drinking alcohol, it's better for you and there's no hangover.

Note: the movement doesn't even have to be strenuous for it to be effective. As basic as it sounds, a walk around a block for five minutes is often enough to reduce or eliminate stress, and therefore eliminate cravings for alcohol. Morning walks in the sunshine put you in a positive mood that stays with you the rest of the day.

Walking barefoot on the grass (a practice known as grounding) is particularly powerful. The Earth generates an electrical pulse known as the Schumann resonance,[60] which is a frequency that has healing and restorative effects on the body. When we walk barefoot on grass, we get connected to that energy and it positively affects our well-being.[61] We feel more connected to nature and the stress easily fades away.

3. THE AMG METHOD FOR KILLING ALCOHOL ANXIETY IN NINETY SECONDS FLAT

Combining gratitude and movement together is a great way to supercharge your results. Here's a simple framework you can use (called the AMG method) to reduce and eliminate alcohol cravings. This works especially well if you're at home and need something to snap you out of a craving ASAP:

1. **Awareness:** Using a notepad or a phone app, record every time you have an intense urge to consume alcohol.
2. **Movement:** Instead of consuming, pick one exercise you can do immediately and begin doing reps until complete exhaustion (push-ups, bodyweight squats, chin-ups, etc.).
3. **Gratitude:** Afterward, write down three to five reasons why you're grateful you did not drink alcohol.

The AMG method works so well because it creates awareness over how many times throughout the day you're feeling the urge to drink. Oftentimes, lack of awareness leads us down the path of destruction. The more aware you become of your mind, the more control you will have over it.

The exercise component creates a rush of endorphins that will flood your brain with feel-good chemicals while also distracting you from the urge to drink. This creates a positive feedback loop instead of a negative one.

After the energy is expended, you're using the post-workout euphoria to fill your mind with positivity at a time when it's more receptive. This helps to reaffirm why you're making positive changes.

4. RECONNECT WITH MOTHER NATURE

Swiss psychiatrist and psychotherapist Carl Jung once noted: "Whenever we touch nature we get clean. People who have got dirty through too much civilization take a walk in the woods, or a bath in the sea."[62] I couldn't agree more.

We all spend entirely too much time inside in front of screens and I believe our bodies resent us for it. Reconnecting with nature can have a profound impact on your mental health. If you're ever feeling grouchy, agitated, or upset for more than two days in a row, I suggest you spend some time outdoors immediately. Put your toes in the grass, take a swim in a lake, or wrap your arms around a tree and breathe deeply. You'll begin to feel your blood pressure drop almost instantly.

Studies have shown that spending time outdoors reduces stress, boosts mood, and promotes a sense of tranquility. Nature can be a serene antidote to the hustle and bustle of daily life.[63]

Ways to reconnect with nature in your daily life:

» **Plan nature walks:** Take a stroll in a local park, forest, or beach. Feel the fresh air against your skin and take in the natural sights and sounds.
» **Gardening:** Getting your hands in the soil can be incredibly grounding. Plant flowers, herbs, or vegetables and take care of them regularly.
» **Mindful observation:** When outdoors, practice mindfulness by fully engaging your senses—notice the colors, sounds, and scents around you. This practice can deepen your connection with nature.
» **Go on a retreat:** If possible, schedule regular retreats away from city life—camping, hiking, or visiting national parks allows you to unplug and recharge.

By immersing yourself in nature, you remember how small you are in comparison to it all. You'll realize that life's problems are outweighed by its overwhelming beauty.

5. FINDING YOUR CREATIVE OUTLET

I'm a firm believer that most of us are guilty of underestimating our own capabilities. You likely have talents and gifts that you take for granted. You toss them aside. You disrespect them. You probably have creative skills you've spent years building that you forget about completely. I'm challenging you to step out of your comfort zone and commit to developing your creative abilities.

Engaging in creative pursuits provides a fantastic outlet for emotional expression and stress relief. Whether you're painting, writing, playing music, crafting, or doing anything else that brings you joy, creativity allows you to channel thoughts and feelings constructively.

Tips for developing your creative outlets:

» **Identify your interests:** Consider what creative activities excite you. It could be painting, journaling, photography, cooking, or anything you can think of. If you're a multi-passionate person, don't obsess too much. Just pick something you'll have fun doing.
» **Create a dedicated space:** Set up a designated area for your creative activities in your house. Even if it's just a corner of your bedroom, having a physical space can help separate this time from everyday stressors and make it feel more special.
» **Allow yourself to be free:** The goal isn't perfection, but expression. Give yourself permission to create without worrying about the outcome. You don't have to show anybody your work and you're not competing with others.
» **Join a community:** Consider joining local or online groups related to your interests. Engaging with others who are enjoying themselves creatively can be motivating. It's also a great way to make friends with people who share your interests, without using alcohol as a social lubricant.

I think the best part about doing something creative is that it distracts you from your stressors while still allowing you to express emotions, feel empowered, and discover new aspects of yourself. It's a form of personal exploration that can lead to deeper self-understanding.

6. BUILD A ROCK-SOLID SUPPORT SYSTEM

A strong group of friends and allies can be the difference between winning and losing in life. You'll need people who care about you to cheer for you when you succeed and hold you accountable when you fall short of your own goals.

Connecting with friends and loved ones provides emotional comfort and a sense of belonging. When you share your experiences, it lightens the burden and fosters connections that enhance your overall well-being. But this isn't something that comes without effort. You'll have to put some energy into maintaining your support system, especially in an age where everybody is busier and more distracted than ever. It takes a fair amount of intentionality to grow and maintain relationships as an adult, but the ROI is immeasurable.

How to build and maintain your support system:

»   **Reach out:** Make it a habit to reach out and spend time with friends or family, even if it's just through a quick call or text. They'll notice the time you put in.
»   **Schedule regular check-ins:** Plan regular get-togethers, whether they be coffee dates, family dinners, or virtual hangouts, to maintain connections.
»   **Be vulnerable:** Don't hesitate to share your struggles with those you trust. Vulnerability can deepen connections and foster empathy. When you share with others, it gives them permission to do the same with you.
»   **Plan things together:** Joining classes, clubs, or volunteer organizations can help you meet new people and nurture friendships. You're never too old to try something new and you shouldn't be afraid to look silly doing so.

Remember, you're not alone in your stress—so lean on others and allow them to lean on you, too. Cultivating your relationships can alleviate your burdens, providing support with laughter, empathy, and shared experiences.

7. WAKE UP AT THE SAME TIME EVERY DAY

Dr. Michael Breus, renowned sleep expert and author of *The Power of When*, spoke with some of my stop-drinking clients to illustrate the devastating effects of alcohol on sleep. Also known as "The Sleep Doctor," Dr. Breus highlights the significant impact of alcohol on sleep and offers insights on how to improve sleep naturally.

According to Dr. Breus, alcohol negatively affects sleep by disrupting the sleep cycle, particularly the deep sleep stages (stages 3 and 4), which are crucial for physical restoration and immune function.

"Alcohol basically destroys stage three and four sleep,"[64] Breus notes, explaining that this disruption is a primary reason people experience hangovers and feel unrefreshed after consuming alcohol.

Breus also emphasizes that alcohol's impact on REM sleep, the stage where most dreaming occurs, is detrimental. "REM sleep is where we see emotional processing and memory consolidation," he explains. Alcohol interferes with these processes, leading to impaired cognitive and emotional functioning.

To improve sleep without relying on alcohol or other substances, Dr. Breus recommends several natural strategies. One of his key suggestions is maintaining a consistent wake-up time.

"The consistency of the wake-up time is the single most important factor for melatonin production," he advises, stressing that this should be practiced every day, not just on weekdays.

For those struggling with insomnia or waking up in the middle of the night, Breus suggests trying the 4-7-8 breathing technique.

8. THE 4-7-8 BREATHING TECHNIQUE

Breath work and intentional breathing techniques have been around forever. We've known for centuries that the breath is a connection to our physical body, our mental well-being, and our spirituality.

You don't need to get too deep with this—just know that deep breathing exercises can calm the autonomic nervous system, which controls the body's involuntary functions. This reduces your stress levels like an automatic thermostat turning down the temperature in your house.

An easy technique you can use is the 4-7-8 breathing method. This method helps to slow down the heart rate, making it easier to fall asleep.

Here's how it works:

- » Inhale deeply for four seconds.
- » Hold your breath for seven seconds.
- » Exhale slowly for eight seconds.
- » Repeat for three to five rounds or until you feel calm.

There are numerous studies that indicate simple exercises like this, when done intentionally, can cause physiological changes that include lowered blood pressure and heart rate, and reduced levels of stress hormones in the blood. When we're not stressed, our cravings either reduce in intensity or are eliminated entirely.

9. STAY HYDRATED TO STOP DRINKING

You need to be drinking more water. Period.

Drinking lots of water can help alcohol cravings subside. A National Institutes of Health study recommends drinking at least half your body weight in ounces of water every day. A gallon of water is 128 fluid ounces. That means a 120-pound woman would need to drink at least half a gallon per day—and a 200-pound man would need to drink almost a gallon. In his book *The TB12 Method*, NFL Hall of Fame quarterback Tom Brady revealed he does exactly that.[65]

Also consider the fact that alcohol is a diuretic—it inhibits the production of the hormone that helps the body reabsorb water. That's why a night at the bar has you running to the bathroom to take a leak every thirty minutes. When you're drinking alcohol, you are losing more water than normal along with electrolytes like sodium, potassium, and magnesium that go with it. Most people who drink are in a constant state of dehydration, even if they don't know it.

Water is like oil to a gas engine. It keeps everything lubricated and running smoothly. It regulates internal temperature, transports nutrients to your joints, and even acts as a shock absorber for vital organs.

Drinking mineral-rich water by adding a pinch of sea salt is even better. You could even add a little honey, maple syrup, or coconut water. This will rehydrate the cells and flush toxins from the liver that accumulate from stress, alcohol, and bad food.

10. NUTRITION AND SUPPLEMENTATION

Can alcohol cravings be conquered with food and supplements?

Julia Ross, a leading expert in nutritional therapy for mood, cravings, and addiction, believes they can. As the author of *The Craving Cure*, *The Mood Cure*, and *The Diet Cure*, Ross shared her expertise on the *Alcohol-Free Lifestyle* podcast, offering groundbreaking insights into how nutrition can play a pivotal role in overcoming alcohol addiction.

Ross argues that nutritional therapy can restore the brain's neurotransmitter balance, significantly reducing cravings without the need for traditional 12-step programs or rehab[66]. She cites the work of Dr. Kenneth Blum, who discovered a strong link between neurotransmitter imbalances and alcoholism. Dr. Blum's research highlights how restoring brain chemistry with amino acids and proper nutrition provides a natural, effective alternative to traditional addiction treatments.

By combining nutrient therapies with a structured diet and supplements, Ross asserts that individuals can give their brains the support they need to heal and thrive, reducing the grip of alcohol cravings.

Ross recommends a diet rich in animal-based proteins, fruits, vegetables, and healthy fats. Additionally, she highlights the following five amino acids as key players in restoring neurotransmitter balance and reducing cravings:

5 KEY AMINO ACIDS FOR REDUCING CRAVINGS

1. **Tyrosine** is known to boost dopamine levels, improving focus and energy. Use with caution, it's not recommended for individuals on mood-related medications, as it may interact.
2. **GABA** has been shown to calm the nervous system and reduce stress-related cravings.
3. **DPA/DLPA (DL-Phenylalanine)** plays a role in retaining natural endorphins, fostering feelings of happiness and pain relief. Alcohol and sugary foods temporarily boost endorphins, offering "comfort" but creating unsustainable cycles. This can help sustain the natural high of endorphins without the negative side effects of alcohol.
4. **Glutamine** supports neurotransmitter function by providing glucose to the brain, helping to stabilize energy and mood.
5. **Tryptophan or 5-HT** is known to aid in serotonin production, alleviating depression, irritability, and negative thoughts. This amino acid is found in animal proteins; plant proteins contain minimal amounts. A word of caution here: it may not be suitable for individuals on certain prescription medications.

As with any changes to diet and supplementation, be sure to consult with your physician before making any changes. These are general findings, not recommendations or prescriptions.

MORE NUTRITIONAL STRATEGIES TO CRUSH CRAVINGS

Dr. Brooke Scheller, a clinical nutrition expert and author of *How to Eat to Change How You Drink*,[67] also shared actionable strategies for reducing cravings during her appearance on the *Alcohol-Free Lifestyle* podcast. Scheller agrees with Ross that nutrition and supplementation can play a vital role in breaking free from alcohol dependence. Her key tips include the following:

Tip #1: Increase Your Protein Intake

Higher protein stabilizes blood sugar, preventing energy highs and lows that can trigger cravings. Incorporate beef, chicken, fish, eggs, cheese and nuts into your diet.

Tip #2: Eat Healthy Fats and Omega-3-Rich Foods

Fish and other foods containing healthy fats like Omega-3 are known as "brain-boosters" because they support brain health and neurotransmitter function. Include avocados, olive oil, and walnuts in your diet.

You should also consider eating foods that support liver health, including beets, broccoli, cabbage, and kale.

Tip #3. Practice Meal Timing

Eat every three to four hours to stabilize blood sugar levels and avoid crashes that may lead to cravings.

Tip 4. Address Vitamin Deficiencies

B vitamins (especially B1 and B12), vitamin C, vitamin D, magnesium, zinc, and iron are key nutrients that are stripped from your body by alcohol consumption. Make sure to replenish deficiencies caused by alcohol use with targeted supplementation.

RECOMMENDED SUPPLEMENTS

If you're healthy enough to do so, I'd consider one or several adding these supplements to your diet as a way to reduce cravings and get an extra boost that replenishes the nutrients you lose from alcohol:

1. **L-Theanine**: Enhances GABA activity, alleviating anxiety-driven cravings.
2. **L-Glutamine (500 mg)**: Supports neurotransmitter function and stabilizes energy levels.
3. **NAC (N-Acetyl Cysteine)**: Proven to reduce cravings and enhance glutathione levels for detoxification.
4. **Chromium Picolinate**: Helps stabilize blood sugar, reducing spikes and crashes.
5. **Methylated B Vitamin Complex**: Supports brain function and restores key nutrients (B1, B12, and folate).
6. **Omega-3 Fatty Acids**: Essential for overall brain health.
7. **Vitamin D**: Improves mood and immune system function.
8. **Ashwagandha**: Promotes relaxation and reduces stress.
9. **Magnesium**: Enhances sleep quality and calms the nervous system.

Try them and see if you feel a difference. Many of our clients report great results.

***

An alcohol-free lifestyle is like a Choose Your Own Adventure book. There are no strict rules to follow. You get to decide what makes it fun and enjoyable for you.

Ultimately, all you have to do to reduce stress is... pretty much anything other than drinking. Experiment with different things. Maybe it's a swim. Standing in the sun. Phoning a friend. Going for a quick run around the block. Picking up a book.

Remember, you don't really want a drink. You just want to change your state. So change your state without the drink. Soon enough, you won't even feel the desire to drink anymore, even in the most high-stress moments.

DON'T JUST DO IT FOR YOURSELF. DO IT FOR YOUR LEGACY.

Once you know better, you must do better. Alcohol is straight poison so I invite you to stop drinking it. Understanding alcohol's effects on your brain and how it affects your professional performance will allow you to make better decisions about your relationship with it. The journey to an alcohol-free lifestyle is not just about removing a habit; it's also about building new skills en route to becoming the best version of yourself.

Now that you have the full picture of exactly how drinking affects your mind, brain, and performance, it's time to go deeper. In the upcoming chapter, we'll discuss exactly how alcohol could be affecting the DNA of your entire lineage...and how by understanding the science of epigenetics, you can make decisions that have a tremendous ripple effect.

Ready to begin your journey to becoming alcohol-free?
Get tools, support, and free resources at
www.alcoholfreelifestyle.com/resources

KEY TAKEAWAYS

» Alcohol interferes with brain function, slowing learning, decision-making, and mood regulation, which impacts your career and relationships.
» Drinking damages the brain over time, especially the hippocampus, making memory, problem-solving, and focus harder.
» You're not performing at your best while drinking—alcohol is holding you back, even if you don't realize it.

CHAPTER 3 REFLECTION POINTS

Write out the answers to the following prompts in your favorite journal to create simple, concrete action steps for your alcohol-free journey.

Reflection: What physical or mental symptoms have I noticed that may be tied to my alcohol consumption?

Question: What benefits could I experience in my energy, focus, or health by eliminating alcohol from my life?

Next Step: What small change can I make in my daily routine to support my body's recovery from the effects of alcohol?

"I NUMBED MY EMOTIONS FOR SO LONG, NOW IT'S TIME TO FEEL THEM"

By Ron Bourgeois
Real Estate Development
Boston, Massachusetts

I HAD BEEN A DRINKER FOR over forty years before finally quitting in 2023. As a business owner, father of three, and grandfather, I've always considered myself a pit bull in life and business, relentlessly pursuing my goals. But this tenacity didn't serve me well when it came to addressing my drinking problem.

My health was deteriorating, with frequent hangovers and the physical toll of alcohol manifesting in weight gain and fatigue. Emotionally, I felt inauthentic, battling shame and a sense of dishonesty that affected my relationships, especially with my family. I wasn't being all I could be. I knew I wasn't living up to my full potential, and I was definitely doing things that weren't as honest or ethical as they should have been.

My drinking also impacted my wealth, as I often made decisions clouded by alcohol, affecting my business acumen and productivity. I knew it was time for me to make a big change, and I realized I had to fully commit to living alcohol-free.

This decision marked a significant shift in my personal development journey—I began participating actively in a coaching group and embracing vulnerability, which I now see was key to my success. Today, I wake up every day with a renewed sense of purpose. Every day, I wake up and say, "Thank you, God, get after it." My big line is, "Seize the day." It's been wonderful.

I numbed my emotions for so long, and now it's time to feel them. It actually feels good. I might not like it at the moment, but ten minutes later, I feel wonderful because I faced this big challenge and won.

My commitment goes beyond just staying alcohol-free. I work out almost daily, have improved my diet, and reconnected with my family, especially my new grandchild. My son had a baby recently, and I've been able to be there, fully present. I'm also bridging the gap with my stepson, trying to strengthen those relationships. If I were still drinking, I probably wouldn't have cared as much. Now, I'm just trying to love them and be a part of their lives.

CHAPTER 4:

UPGRADE YOUR EPIGENETICS

"Intoxicating drinks have produced evils more deadly, because more continuous, than all those caused to mankind by the great historic scourges of war, famine and pestilence combined."

—WILLIAM GLADSTONE

I N CHAPTER 1, I PRESENTED a study that ranked alcohol as one of the most harmful drugs to communities at large. That's because when you drink, it affects many more people than just yourself. It can affect your lineage.

In this chapter, we delve into the profound and often overlooked realm of epigenetics, exploring how alcohol consumption extends its influence beyond the individual drinker to touch the lives of future generations.

The term *epigenetics* refers to the study of changes in gene expression caused not by alterations in the DNA sequence but by external or environmental factors that switch genes on and off. This emerging field of science offers invaluable insights into how our lifestyle choices, particularly our alcohol consumption, can have long-lasting, multi-generational effects.

During periods of severe stress, like a famine, increases in substance use—including alcohol—are often observed. Alcohol can exacerbate the body's stress response, compounding the effects initiated by other stressors like malnutrition. In the winter of 1944-1945, the Netherlands experienced a severe famine triggered by a German blockade in the final months of World War II known as the Dutch Hunger Winter. This crisis not only led to immediate hardship and suffering, but also provided scientists with a unique window into the long-term health impacts of environmental stress and how adult consumption of alcohol can negatively impact unborn children.

A 2008 study[68] showed that children born during the famine, known as the Hunger Winter babies, exhibited a higher instance of epigenetic changes in their DNA that resulted in serious health consequences later in life—even if they were still in utero during the famine.

These health consequences included:

- » Metabolic disorders such as obesity and Type 2 Diabetes
- » Cardiovascular diseases
- » Mental health disorders such as schizophrenia, depression, and anxiety
- » Reproductive issues
- » Accelerated cognitive decline

Of course, this is all bad news. Let's dive into the fascinating world of epigenetics so that you can learn exactly what's happening at a DNA level to yourself and your offspring when you drink.

EPIGENETICS IN A NUTSHELL

Before you get PTSD from high school biology: epigenetics is the study of how our behaviors and environmental factors can influence gene expression.

You can't change the way your face looks without plastic surgery. But you can change your facial expressions—and that makes a huge difference. Similarly, you can't actually change your genes, but you can change how they express themselves. That expression, for better or worse, can be passed down to future generations.

To understand how your epigenetics are affected by alcohol, let's go over the basics you need to understand about DNA. DNA is the molecule that carries the "instruction manual" for building everything in your body. It consists of two strands in a helix structure.

The DNA strands are very long and that means your body has to pack it very tightly. Each cell in your body contains "over 2 meters of DNA if stretched end-to-end; yet the nucleus of a human cell, which contains the DNA, is only about 6 micrometers (μm) in diameter. This is geometrically equivalent to packing 40 km (24 miles) of extremely fine thread into a tennis ball!"[69]

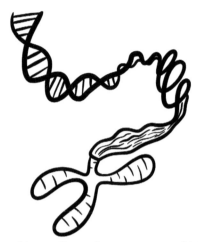

DNA and histones combine to form chromosomes, which are tightly coiled
structures that package genetic material within the nucleus of a cell.

To do this, DNA is combined with proteins called histones.
When the DNA and protein combine, they form protein complexes
called chromatids. As these chromatids condense, they create
chromosomes. You have forty-six chromosomes stored in the
nucleus of your cells, twenty-three from each parent.[70]

Every cell in your body has the same genes inside of it. A
muscle cell, nerve cell and a lung cell all contain the same genetic
code—but because they have different structures and functions in
the body, they only express certain genes. This expression happens when DNA and histones inside the cell are "tagged" by tiny
chemicals that can modify that expression. These tags can turn
certain genes in a cell on or off.

For example, a bone cell will turn on genes that are important
for bone growth and turn off genes important for lung function.
Conversely, lung cells will turn off genes for bone growth and turn
on genes important for lung function. The prefix epi- comes from
the Greek word for "above," so epigenetic modifications are literally changes happening "above the genes." Imagine a little worker
hovering above each gene and flipping the "on" or "off" switch for
different characteristics depending on what's needed in specific
cells. Those are epigenetic modifications.

On a practical level, we've all heard the "nature" (genetics) versus "nurture" (environment) debate when it comes to early childhood development. The common consensus is that both factors both play a pivotal role. But what role do epigenetic modifications play in human development?

HOW EPIGENETIC DAMAGE
FROM ALCOHOL IMPACTS YOUR CHILDREN

Most people know that drinking during pregnancy is bad for fetal development. When a mother exposes a fetus to alcohol during pregnancy, it predisposes the unborn child to a wide range of health problems, such as Fetal Alcohol Spectrum Disorders (FASD)—which can create learning disabilities, behavioral challenges, neurological damage, and even physical abnormalities.[71]

However, most people aren't aware that even drinking before pregnancy can affect unborn children by modifying maternal epigenetics, thereby altering the quality of the egg.[72] As a result, even if a mother does not drink during pregnancy, her eggs may carry epigenetic modifications that can affect her children.

Have you ever compared the yolk of a farm fresh, cage-free organic chicken egg to that of a factory farmed egg from the grocery store? The organic yolk will have a much deeper amber color and a much richer taste than its factory farmed counterpart. That's because the stress of being cooped up and fed crappy food affects the quality of the product. It's the same with humans.

Lest we pick on moms too much, it's important to note that paternal use of alcohol can alter sperm epigenetics as well. For example, paternal alcohol consumption has been linked to changes in DNA that may disrupt gene expression critical for brain development in the child.

Additionally, a father's diet significantly impacts the DNA in sperm. Research has shown that high-fat diets or nutritional deficiencies can lead to damaged or lowered sperm count, which can impact offspring metabolism, growth, and development. An unhealthy diet, which is highly correlated with regular alcohol consumption, can influence genes associated with obesity and metabolic syndrome in children.

It would be reason enough to stop drinking if it were only your epigenetics being affected. Many parents would probably hope their kids would adopt a "Do as I say, not as I do" strategy for life and make smart choices. However, epigenetic changes mean that the choices you make for yourself may impact your kids negatively before they're even born. Here are some examples of the "second-order" epigenetic consequences that alcohol use disorder can have on offspring.[73]

1. **Behavioral and emotional regulation alterations:** Children of parents with a history of AUD may exhibit altered behavioral patterns, including heightened anxiety levels, depression, or increased impulsivity.

2. **Increased susceptibility to substance use disorders:** Epigenetic alterations can affect neurobiological pathways associated with addiction, increasing the likelihood that offspring will develop alcohol-related problems.[74]

3. **Impaired stress response:** Lifelong exposure to stress, particularly in the context of trauma and alcohol use within families, can lead to dysregulation of the hormonal response to stress, making future generations more reactive to environmental stressors.[75]

4. **Development of chronic health issues:** Epigenetic changes can predispose children to chronic health problems, including obesity, diabetes, and cardiovascular diseases, influenced by the health and lifestyle choices of their ancestors.

5. **Mental health disorders:** The intergenerational transmission of mental health disorders in families with a history of addiction can manifest as increased rates of depression, anxiety disorders, or PTSD.[76]

6. **Resistance to treatment and recovery:** Epigenetic changes may foster a reluctance to engage in recovery or treatment modalities, as inherited patterns might lead individuals to distrust support systems or believe that they are inherently predisposed to addiction.[77]

If you're someone who comes from a family with a history of heavy drinking or you're a parent who is worried about how your use of alcohol will affect the epigenetics of your family, this all paints a very gloomy picture. But don't despair. The good news is that changes in your lifestyle can give you considerable control over your epigenetic destiny.

SEVEN FACTORS THAT IMPACT YOUR EPIGENETIC DESTINY

If your parents or grandparents had an alcohol use disorder, does that mean you will develop one as well? Well, according to popular research, the answer is yes. You have a 50 percent increased risk of developing AUD yourself if close relatives also suffer from it, according to the National Institute of Alcohol Abuse and Alcoholism. BUT... just because that's the case, it doesn't mean you have to allow those epigenetics to control your destiny.

The biggest levers you have to overcome the negative effects of alcohol on your DNA are behavioral. You can alter your chances of developing AUD by simply changing your environment and making lifestyle choices. It's not your fault that you have a higher risk of developing AUD due to your family history, but it is your responsibility to do something about it. If you've ever excused your drinking with, "Alcoholism runs in my family," you've used an unfortunate truth to create an easy out for yourself. Stop defending your alcohol consumption. Stop defining your habits by those of your parents. Be one hundred percent responsible for your health.

If instead of focusing on your family history, you focus your energy on changing the things you can control in the present, you'll have a much greater chance at success—no matter what bad habits run in your family. I've listed seven specific factors below that impact your epigenetic expression. We have discussed some of them in previous chapters, but it's worth looking at them from an epigenetic lens here. When monitored and improved, these epigenetic levers can help heal the damage caused to your DNA by the drinking habits of yourself or your parents. This is how you take back control of your epigenetics.

EPIGENETIC FACTOR #1: DIET AND NUTRITION

They say that you are what you eat because the content of your diet, how much you eat and when you eat all play a role in gene expression. This also includes proper hydration and supplementation.[78]

Action step: One of the simplest steps you can take to have more control over your epigenetics as it relates to nutrition is simply tracking what you eat. Management guru Peter Drucker was known to have famously said "what gets measured gets managed"—and that applies to food, too. The simple act of writing down what you're eating and when will bring more awareness to what you're consuming and allow you to make better choices. There are many helpful apps like MyFitnessPal which will log all your food and even give you healthy recipes as well.

EPIGENETIC FACTOR #2: EXERCISE

How often you move is the most important factor. Cardiovascular fitness, strength, flexibility and mobility routines can all contribute to positive epigenetic changes.[79]

Action step: Make daily movement a non-negotiable in your life. You may not have the time (or desire) to workout at a gym. That's fine. Start with setting a step count for yourself every day and try to maintain or beat your best number on a daily basis. About 5,000 steps per day is a good place to start—then do your best to never miss a day. This process will likely help you drop a few pounds, but that's not really the point. The downstream positive effects of this habit for your mobility, metabolism and mental health can create a cascade of benefits that improve your gene expression.

EPIGENETIC FACTOR #3: MENTAL HEALTH

Your self-perception, internal dialogue and mental state all create the context for your mental health, which has a huge epigenetic impact. You can turn genes on or off through thought alone.[80]

Action step: We've mentioned meditation, prayer, mindfulness, and breath work routines already in this book. They are not just passing trends. I highly recommend you experiment with them for epigenetic reasons.

Clinical research shows that practices like meditation can create feelings of joy, gratitude, and love. In turn, these feelings can induce heart coherence[81]—a state characterized by a stable, ordered heart rhythm. This coherent state is associated with enhanced cognitive function, emotional stability, and greater resilience to stress, which all have positive epigenetic implications.

EPIGENETIC FACTOR #4: HORMONAL BALANCE

Hormones are chemical messengers produced by different glands in your body and transported through your bloodstream. Hormones like cortisol, insulin, estrogen, and testosterone play significant roles in how your genes express themselves. Whether due to natural life stages (like puberty or menopause), stress, or endocrine-disrupting chemicals, hormonal changes can influence your epigenetics big time.[82]

Action step: your hormone balance is something that you can have an impact on through diet, exercise and sleep—though you'll never have direct control. One of the best ways you can take responsibility for your hormonal balance is to get regular blood tests by a qualified physician.

Understanding what your normal levels are for important markers like testosterone, estrogen, insulin and thyroid hormones can give you a good baseline for knowing when things aren't right. From there, you can take appropriate steps with your doctor. Most people only take blood tests when there's a problem—but making time for your health while you're still feeling good and being proactive rather than reactive will keep you healthy.

EPIGENETIC FACTOR #5: SOCIAL ENVIRONMENT

In the years since the pandemic, studies have given more visibility to what researchers are calling the "loneliness epidemic." Loneliness has been linked to increased risks of anxiety, depression, heart disease, cognitive decline, and even premature death.[83] Having a strong support network of family, friends, and colleagues can influence gene expression that combat chronic health issues related to isolation.

Action step: as we get older, we get more locked into our life and work routines. It can be harder to form new friendships or nurture existing ones because we're so busy. Resist the urge to put your head down and work yourself to death. Make an effort to see friends and family. It won't always be convenient, but it will do wonders for your mental and emotional health.

One simple step you can take is finding a "third space." If you spend most of your time at home and in the office, a third space is a place for recreation where you can break out of the routine, connect with likeminded people and relax. For some, this means signing up for a group fitness program at the gym, an art class at your local community college or even a volunteer project. Your third space should allow you to develop more social connections, learn about yourself and let your hair down. Don't isolate yourself. Make an effort to put yourself in places where you're bound to connect with others and the stress relief will do wonders for your epigenetic expression.

EPIGENETIC FACTOR #6: SLEEP PATTERNS

Consistent, high-quality sleep is crucial for maintaining healthy gene expression. Alcohol consumption disrupts both REM sleep and deep sleep, which are responsible for cognitive function and physical recovery, respectively. Disrupted sleep patterns can lead to changes in the expression of genes involved in metabolism, stress response, and immune function.[84]

Action step: Create a sleep routine that guarantees high-quality sleep each night. Here are some of the things I've tried that have helped:

> » **Keep a consistent schedule:** Go to bed at the same time every night, even on weekends. This will get you into a consistent rhythm.
> » **Kill the screens:** No screens at least one hour before bed. Bright blue lights from LED screens trick your brain into thinking it's still daytime, delaying the release of melatonin, the hormone which tells your body it's time to sleep. If you choose to ignore my advice and continue with screens at night anyway, invest in a quality pair of orange-lens blue-blocking glasses, such as Swannies from my sleep company, Swanwick Sleep.
> » **Loosen up:** Do some gentle stretching and deep breathing before getting into bed as a way of relaxing your body and nervous system.

» **Wind down:** Use a diffuser with essential oils like lavender as well as soothing music to help yourself wind down.

EPIGENETIC FACTOR #7: GUT MICROBIOME

Healthy bacteria in your gut microbiome help to regulate your immune system. You can strengthen your microbiome through diet and supplementation. Alcohol weakens it.[85] Scientists are only now beginning to understand the full impact of the microbiome on overall health. The microbial communities in other parts of the body (like the skin and mouth) also interact with your body and can influence gene expression locally and systemically.[86]

Action step: To support a healthy gut microbiome, focus on incorporating a diverse diet rich in fruits, vegetables, and whole grains, which promotes beneficial bacteria. Include probiotic-rich foods like yogurt, kefir, sauerkraut, and kimchi to introduce helpful microbes into your system. Limiting sugar and processed foods is also important, as they can disrupt the balance of gut flora. Finally, staying well-hydrated helps maintain a healthy digestive system and supports overall gut health.

PULLING IT ALL TOGETHER

Your environment and lifestyle choices are continuously interacting with your genome, and that affects your gene expression. There are no hard rules when it comes to epigenetic modification and gene expression amongst people. It's complex, and the difficulty is we cannot always say for sure which factors turn which genes on and off.

You cannot be totally certain which elements of your behaviors or environment are affecting your epigenetics. The exact mechanisms of how environmental factors lead to specific epigenetic changes are still being studied. You also cannot say for sure which of your epigenetic traits or gene expressions you will pass on to your offspring. The only thing you can do is to appreciate the profound connection between your environment, behavior, and genome. You must respect the role epigenetics play in your life, while also recognizing that your behaviors, not your family history, are the key to making lasting changes around alcohol.

Start by understanding the seven factors above—and commit to making your first epigenetic improvement by quitting alcohol. This is the lead domino that will make everything else easier. By changing your behavior and improving your own epigenetics, you're opening the door for future generations to change and improve in positive ways as well.

And speaking of future generations: the next chapter is all about how your new alcohol-free lifestyle will open up the door to career fulfillment and incredible wealth. See you there.

Ready to begin your journey to becoming alcohol-free?
Get tools, support, and free resources at
www.alcoholfreelifestyle.com/resources

KEY TAKEAWAYS

» Alcohol alters your genes, increasing the risk of addiction, mental health issues, and chronic diseases—even for future generations.
» Quitting alcohol doesn't just improve your health—it helps break cycles of genetic predisposition to addiction and disease in your family.
» Your choices shape your genes—quitting alcohol, improving diet, exercise, and sleep can rewire your biology for a healthier future.

CHAPTER 4 REFLECTION POINTS

Write out the answers to the following prompts in your favorite journal to create simple, concrete action steps for your alcohol-free journey.

Reflection: How has alcohol use potentially impacted my long-term health or the legacy I want to leave for my family?

Question: If I could pass down one healthy habit to the next generation, what would it be, and why?

Next Step: What is one daily action I can take today to improve my health and epigenetic expression?

"LIFE GETS TO BE FUN AGAIN. MY SOUL CAN BREATHE."

By Jessica Gaines
Real Estate Broker
Louisville, Kentucky

STOPPED DRINKING WITH PROJECT 90 in 2018. Back then I was caught in a cycle of drinking to unwind and relying on stimulants to power through my demanding days. I felt like I was in quicksand up to my neck, filled with shame, isolation, and exhaustion. My marriage was ending, and I felt utterly drained. I was just surviving rather than thriving, with feelings of complete isolation and loneliness. I felt ashamed of how much I was drinking.

When I quit drinking, I began to focus on life's possibilities rather than what I was giving up. This shift in perspective opened my eyes to the endless opportunities that had been obscured by my alcohol use. Now, I enjoy deeper connections, better emotional control, and a renewed zest for life.

I've slimmed down and feel more toned. My complexion is clearer, and I feel like I have blood and rosiness in my cheeks. Even my hair is better. These changes reflect not only my physical transformation but also my overall sense of vitality.

This was just the beginning of my journey, and I am a completely different person now. My life feels like a complete exhale; I no longer have to tap out or numb myself from it. I am consistently reaching new levels of surrender, relaxation, receptivity, devotion, and discipline to live the life of my dreams in ways I truly never thought were possible. Life gets to be fun. My soul can breathe.

I no longer even think about drinking. My life has expanded in ways I hadn't imagined—I'm motivated at work, considering adoption, traveling, and continually discovering new passions. Becoming alcohol-free has profoundly impacted my life.

CHAPTER 5:

HOW ELIMINATING ALCOHOL GROWS YOUR BUSINESS AND YOUR WEALTH

"Some of the domestic evils of drunkenness are houses without windows, gardens without fences, fields without tillage, barns without roofs, children without clothing, principles, morals, or manners."

—BENJAMIN FRANKLIN

I RECALL BEING AT A BUSINESS dinner in London in August 2019 at the Edition Hotel in the swanky suburb of Fitzrovia. The dinner was hosted by my first business mentor Tai Lopez, an investor, online influencer and marketing expert. There were eighteen of us at the dinner table. How many of us drank alcohol? Zero. Peak performers don't need alcohol to socialize, have a good time or do business. No alcohol needed, no alcohol consumed.

Almost everyone at the table was generating at least six figures in their business, and many were generating exponentially more than that. And yet nobody drank. We talked business, some made deals, and all made new friendships or strengthened existing ones. We had a good time, shared ideas and stories, made new connections, and supported one another. It was clear that no one gave a second thought to the absence of fancy cocktails or expensive bottles of wine around the table.

Incidentally, I gave a sixty-minute talk at the dinner on how to build multimillion-dollar businesses through relationships, healthy habits, and helping people. One of the habits I presented was the choice to go alcohol-free for life. In this case, I was preaching to the converted.

As I shared around the dinner table that night, most peak performers I know and associate with either don't drink at all or drink rarely. That's because they know what I know: that alcohol is the biggest productivity killer around. That it's a slow sap of our energy, focus, and potential that offers little or nothing in return. From six- and seven-figure entrepreneurs to Hollywood stars to pro athletes, the pattern is undeniable: Those who are at the top of their game don't have a place for alcohol in their daily lives.

In other words: alcohol is an investment with no possibility of making your money back.

When I quit drinking alcohol in 2010, I had no entrepreneurial experience. I'd always had jobs working for someone else. But with my newfound clarity and drive, I decided to dive into the business world. Soon after, I created two seven-figure businesses: a health-and-performance coaching business, Alcohol-Free Lifestyle, and a sleep products company, Swanwick Sleep.

I squandered money for years when I drank, only to generate millions when I quit. Certainly, quitting alcohol isn't the only factor in my success—but it was the biggest domino in a chain of positive habit changes. I credit being alcohol-free with giving me the clarity and focus and confidence to achieve business success—and I have heard the same sentiment expressed by countless other entrepreneurs and business leaders.

This chapter will take a closer look at exactly how alcohol kills your professional productivity, with a specific focus on the money you're losing by continuing to drink.

The facts are just as terrifying as they are enlightening.

ALCOHOL: THE ULTIMATE PROFESSIONAL PRODUCTIVITY KILLER

In previous chapters, we looked at the science behind what alcohol does to your brain, thinking processes, and productivity. We saw that it slows down the brain's ability to process information and can impact higher-order cognitive abilities, including impairing the ability to synthesize different thoughts required for abstract and logical reasoning as well as social intelligence and decision-making. These effects are particularly damaging for entrepreneurs, high performers, and professionals who depend on being razor sharp to succeed in a fast-paced work world.

Research shows that one of the keys to productivity and effective decision-making is the trait of cognitive adaptability,[87] which organizational psychologists define as "the ability to effectively and appropriately evolve or adapt decision policies (i.e., to learn) given feedback (inputs) from the environmental context in which cognitive processing is embedded." In simple language, it's your brain's ability to adapt to change.

Entrepreneurial success has more to do with nimble adaptation of one's business concept than it does with having the right concept from the outset or "being in the right place at the right time." To be clear, this doesn't just apply to entrepreneurs and founders. It's my conviction that we all need to approach our careers and professional lives with an entrepreneurial mindset, regardless of whether or not we actually launch our own business. In today's business climate, that kind of innovative thinking and quick adaptability is a requirement for success, whether you're a salesperson, a manager, or a CFO.

You have to be able to respond strategically and creatively to changes in your business environment. You need to cultivate a mindset that supports adaptive decision-making. The first step to doing that is to become aware of and address anything that might be getting in the way, whether it's high stress levels, a regular drinking habit, a fear of failure, or anything else. Ask yourself honestly: *How quickly am I able to adapt to changing circumstances? What's slowing me down?* Consider the non-beneficial habits and the obstacles (both internal and external) that keep you from thinking and acting quickly, confidently, and creatively.

In order to achieve ambitious goals in business, you need to perform at your best—but you can't do that if you're being weighed down by the heavy yoke of alcohol. I often reference Nassim Nicholas Taleb's concept of "perficiendi via negativa"—performance by removal. To make a car faster, remove extra weight. That makes sense to me.

With many of my clients and colleagues in the business world, I've seen that regular alcohol consumption is a non-beneficial habit that can become, over time, a significant obstacle to adaptability. And here's the thing: once someone removes that layer of clouding that drinking creates, they tend to get much more clear on all the other obstacles. It's not just the removal of alcohol that accelerates your business—it's the mental bandwidth returned to you in alcohol's absence that allows you to increase your capacity to do impactful work.

With the enhanced energy and clarity that comes with sobriety, you're not only able to see clearly what else is getting in the way of peak performance, but you also have the focus and resolve to tackle each of those obstacles. It's a double win. It's like losing fat and gaining muscle at the same time.

By the way, this isn't just me preaching from the alcohol-free pulpit. Some of the most successful entrepreneurs in the world—including Warren Buffet, Elon Musk, Jack Dorsey, Oprah Winfrey, and Sara Blakely—rarely drink or have completely cut out alcohol altogether. It's inspiring to see.

Despite all the evidence to the contrary, you may still be of the opinion that you can do your best work while maintaining a regular drinking habit. Many of my "Type A" professional clients are stubborn. In that case, let me speak to you in a language you'll understand better.

"In business, I've learned it's better to solve a small problem early than to let it grow into a big one," said one of our *Project 90* clients. "That's why I'm here—before it's too late." This book is your opportunity to solve the problem before it's too late.

Let's talk about how much your drinking habit is costing you financially.

CALCULATING THE FINANCIAL TOLL OF ALCOHOL

Let's take a cold, hard look at the numbers.

Your current drinking habits are likely costing you at least $100,000 per year. Millions over the course of your career. Yes, you read that correctly. Whether you're an entrepreneur or corporate executive or top performer in your organization, you're likely leaving at least \$100K a year of revenue or income on the table. Don't believe it? I didn't believe it either, for a while. And then I took a good look at the math. What I unearthed was both frightening and exciting at the same time.

In a moment, I'm going to invite you to take my Alcohol Lost Money Calculator test. We're going to determine the actual financial cost of your drinking habits. What I've found is that it's not the money you spend on alcohol that costs you hundreds of thousands of dollars. It's the money you don't make because of alcohol. That's called "opportunity cost."

As you already know, alcohol (even in small doses) has numerous detrimental effects on your physical and mental health. If you have only one drink a night each night of the week, the toxins will stay in your body for seven days. This will likely mean:

» You don't sleep as well
» You wake up irritable
» Your energy levels are low
» You're less productive
» You lose your edge
» You make poor decisions

If this tracks with your personal experience, you won't be surprised to learn that research in the *Journal of Occupational and Environmental Medicine* found employees with alcohol dependence had higher rates of absenteeism and were less productive compared to their alcohol-free counterparts.[88] A similar study in *Addiction* indicated that workers who frequently consumed alcohol were at an increased risk for job turnover and lower career achievement, suggesting that cutting back or quitting alcohol can have a positive impact on professional growth.[89]

Consider your workday following a night of drinks. Do you often feel tired at the end of the day? Maybe, because you feel tired, you don't do a deal you ordinarily would have. Maybe, because you're lacking focus and motivation, you only push 70 percent instead of 90 percent.

It all adds up over time. It's the sales call you don't make or the project you keep putting on the back burner because you're lethargic and foggy. Those opportunities in your life are your sacrifices at the altar of alcohol.

Let's determine how much money this habit is actually costing you. For a moment, forget the amount of money you spend on alcohol and alcohol-related activities. We'll come back to that. First, let's calculate how much money you might be leaving on the table. You can do it easily in just three steps.

The Alcohol Lost Money Calculator:

1. With your drinking habits the way they are, how much revenue did you generate in your job or business last year?
2. If you were consistently alcohol-free and enjoyed a clearer mind, more energy, less stress, extra motivation, and laser focus, how much revenue do you think could you generate this year?
3. Subtract (1) from (2)

Whatever number you arrive at in Step 3, that's what your drinking is potentially costing you in lost revenue each year. Look at it. Think about it evaporating from your wallet. Imagine a $100,000 investment portfolio going to zero instantly. Every time you drink, that's what it's costing you. That's money you're NOT generating. You're leaving it on the table.

It's a simple process, but it does require a certain amount of self-reflection and self-awareness. You need to get really clear and honest with yourself about your current energy levels and performance, and what you know you'd be capable of if you took the energy that's getting drained by your drinking habit and redirected it into your business.

HOW TO MAKE AN EXTRA $100,000
THIS YEAR BY GOING ALCOHOL-FREE

Let's make it a little more concrete. As an example, think about a real estate broker, John, who currently generates around $180K a year. John is a social drinker. He has a glass or two of wine each day to take the edge off. He attends real estate broker networking events once a month where he has a few drinks. He plays golf on the weekends with friends and enjoys a couple of beers after the round. John is not an alcoholic. He's considered a normal drinker. John sells an average of one residential property per month, making around $15K in commissions. John makes $180K a year from those twelve sales. Not bad.

Other people might think John is crushing it, but John knows he's not performing anywhere close to his full potential. His nightly drink or two of red wine leaves him feeling sluggish most mornings. That means he doesn't make as many prospecting calls in the morning as he knows he probably should. Later in the afternoon, John starts to feel foggy. The last thirty minutes of his workday is not really work. He knows he's drifting along. Those thirty minutes are critical. John could be speaking to another prospect or meeting another client or closing another deal. The devil is in the details. It's not one sluggish day or missed lead that's dragging him down, it's the aggregate effect over time. It's the negative compound interest of a bad habit.

If John stopped drinking, slept better and had the energy to make even just a few additional calls, it's not unrealistic to suggest that he could shift from feeling like a 6/10 to a 9/10. With that additional clarity, focus and energy, John could make at least one additional sale every two months or six additional sales per year. At an average of $15,000 commission per sale, John can now generate an additional $90K a year in income. (Six more sales = 6 × $15K commission = $90K additional revenue.)

Because John is now alcohol-free, he's no longer spending the $10K a year he was spending buying alcohol. With the added revenue, he's now $100K better off. This is a simplified example meant to illustrate the hidden financial impact of a seemingly negligible bad habit over time.

Time Period	Opportunity Cost	Alcohol Expense	Related Expenses	Total Invested	Total Lost (Assuming 5% Interest)
1 year	$90,000	$10,000	$5,000	$105,000	$110,250
5 years	$450,000	$50,000	$25,000	$525,000	$609,200
10 years	$900,000	$100,000	$50,000	$1,050,000	$1,386,712
40 years	$3,600,000	$400,000	$200,000	$4,200,000	$13,318,175

Table 5.1: Alcohol Lost Money Table

If you think $100,000 is a lot to lose over alcohol, Table 5.1 shows how much John stands to lose up to $13 MILLION over the next few decades if he continues on the exact same trajectory. Are you beginning to see the real cost of your drinking habits? How much are you leaving on the table?

Maybe the number isn't $100,000 for you at your current level of earning. Maybe it's $15,000—which could be enough to make a difference in your quality of life or your ability to invest in a new business venture. In a single year, that number could amount to a modest overall improvement in your life. Over five years, it could mean that you're able to successfully launch a new venture or buy a home when you wouldn't otherwise have been able to. That's how this one small change adds up in ways that truly transform your life.

Here's another example, this one from a client of mine, Amy, who owned an interior design company in Boston. Amy told me she tripled her business within ninety days of quitting drinking. When Amy was drinking on a daily basis, she said she was distracted and irritable with herself and colleagues. After giving up alcohol, she felt clear and energized. She attracted more clients and was able to be more present with them, which translated into several lucrative referrals. Clients love talking to people who are on the ball. Colleagues notice a real difference, tempers are less frayed and a relaxed calm takes over. The seemingly minor shifts in Amy's mood and demeanor quickly translated into tangible results.

Another client, Nicole, was a former daily drinker from Seattle who suspected that her habit was contributing to her chronic, low-level depression. Nicole came to me complaining that she felt stuck. When she stopped drinking, she said she generated clarity and focus, increased energy and happiness levels. She also quit her job that was "depleting my soul", started an argan oil business and produced international retreats for nurses. She says she feels happier and more fulfilled than she's ever felt.

In each of these cases, it's not just quitting alcohol that creates meaningful life and business improvements. It's the increased bandwidth gained after quitting drinking that provided them with the runway to do their best work. With the newfound clarity of sobriety, you'll be able to work harder for longer. You'll be able to learn new skills more quickly. You'll be able to adapt more readily to changing market conditions and make better decisions. Those are the real needle movers—quitting alcohol just removes the roadblocks.

If you quit drinking but don't do anything with the newfound energy, you won't see noticeable improvements in your professional life. But if you focus your new energy into making incremental shifts, they'll quickly add up to real results. Don't discount the potential bottom-line impact of bringing a compounded 10 percent more energy, focus, and clarity to your work each day.

UNPACKING THE TOTAL COST OF DRINKING

I said earlier that we'd talk about what you spend on alcohol. I think this cost is mostly inconsequential compared with the lost opportunity cost. But it's a fascinating study to look at the math here, too. It's just another example of how alcohol's slow drain can add up to a significant cost (financial, mental, and otherwise) over time.

There's no denying that alcohol is expensive. It's especially expensive in bars and restaurants, which is where most people drink, most of the time. The costs add up over time. According to several recent studies, moderate drinking is defined as up to one drink per day for women and up to two drinks per day for men.[90] Thirty to sixty drinks per month being labeled as "moderate" is insanity to me, but I digress.

If you're looking at $10 plus tip per drink (in cities like LA, London, and New York, it's going to be a lot more), that means you're spending nearly $100 a week on alcohol. That means $400 per month spent on alcohol, or almost $5,000 a year—and that's for only one drink a day. For men, at two drinks per day, we're talking $10,000 or more per year.

Even if you're buying alcohol in bulk and drinking at home, it still adds up. A liter of alcohol at a time, which can generate about eight drinks if you use four ounces of liquor per drink, can cost between $20 and $40. If you need two liters of alcohol to get you through the week, then that's still between $40 and $80 that you're spending per week. When wine or scotch is the alcohol of choice, the cost is even higher. It's estimated that it costs around $800 a month—or $10,000 a year—to support a heavy drinker's wine habit.

How much is your drinking habit costing you?
Visit www.alcoholfreelifestyle.com/scorecard to take our online quiz and find out exactly how much you're leaving on the table.

Feeling courageous? Take a moment to crunch your own numbers, adding up what you spend for drinks both at home and out on the town—and be sure to factor in tax and tip. By themselves, a few beers or a bottle of wine probably won't cost you more than $30. But when you drink daily, or even weekly, the costs compound over time.

Poor financial decisions often accompany drinking, too. Do you have to take a day off work because you're tired or hungover?

There's a financial cost to that. Do you buy cold and flu tablets at the pharmacy because you've run down your immune system from excessive drinking? Do you take an Uber or taxi home when buzzed? More expenditure. Are you out to dinner and ordering dessert or shouting rounds at the bar? There's more money and more tax to pay there. It goes on and on.

Consider the average cost of each drink, the average number of drinks consumed, the average number of drinks you buy for others, and the number of days. Then add up the alcohol-related costs. Most people who drink regularly will be shocked at the amount of cash they spend on alcohol directly or on alcohol-adjacent expenses.

Researchers from Cardiff University and Oxford studying the long-term effects of alcohol looked at the cost of drinking from a more holistic vantage point. Examining the impact of alcohol consumption on health, mental ability, and relationships, they found that regular drinking "reduces our health, happiness, employability and our ability to think and remember."[91]

They also concluded that, for long-term drinkers, each weekly bottle of wine is equivalent to $3,100 a year in damage to health and quality of life. At one bottle of wine per week, that adds up to over $150,000 per year in damage to your health. The research, funded by the Medical Research Council, focused on 141,000 British drinkers between the ages of thirty-seven and seventy-three. It found that, besides the "adverse cognitive impact" of alcohol, it also leads to higher risks of depression and insomnia—both massive productivity (and revenue) killers.

Money—like time and energy—is a currency. How are you spending the currency that's available to you? Are you being intentional in your expenditure? Are you putting your time, energy and money toward things that will give you a good return on investment in terms of your health, quality of life, and career success? Or are you investing in things that ultimately come at a cost in all of these areas?

One of the big wake-up calls for many people when they quit drinking is seeing how empowering it is to take all the resources that were previously being siphoned into their drinking habit and redirect them toward more meaningful, high-ROI investment.

What do you really want to create in your life? If you have big goals, you'll be able to achieve them much more easily with the time, energy and financial resources you'll gain from giving up drinking. I guarantee that once you embrace the alcohol-free lifestyle and begin seeing how much power you can pour into your career, you'll never look back.

So far, we've looked at all the different ways that quitting alcohol will benefit you personally and professionally. In the next chapter we're going to take a deep dive into exactly how changing your habits around alcohol will lead to the most fulfilling relationships you've ever had. You'll even get "scripts" for talking with friends, family, significant others and coworkers about your decision to quit.

Ready to begin your journey to becoming alcohol-free?
Get tools, support, and free resources at
www.alcoholfreelifestyle.com/resources

KEY TAKEAWAYS

» Drinking is very expensive — it costs more than money, lowers productivity, slows decision-making and threatens career opportunities.
» Living alcohol-free is a competitive edge, sharpening your adaptability, creativity and strategic thinking.
» Quitting alcohol frees up time, money, and energy, giving you a massive return on investment in life and business.

CHAPTER 5 REFLECTION POINTS

Write out the answers to the following prompts in your favorite journal to create simple, concrete action steps for your alcohol-free journey.

Reflection: How has alcohol impacted my productivity, decision-making, or ability to achieve my professional goals?

Question: What could I accomplish in my career or finances with the time and energy I currently spend on drinking?

Next Step: What is one professional goal I can set that reflects the clarity and focus I want to gain from being alcohol-free?

"I RECLAIMED MY LIFE AFTER A FORTY-YEAR DRINKING HABIT"

By Steve Wilt
Institutional Financial Advisor
Akron, Ohio

I RECLAIMED MY LIFE AFTER A forty-year drinking habit. My journey to an alcohol-free life began with a growing realization that something was amiss. Despite my outward success in my firm, being a dedicated family man, a community leader, and an avid golfer and tennis player, I felt like I was living in a "self-imposed prison." At times, I felt like an imposter.

I remember the moment it all became clear: It was during a session with our Alcohol-Free Lifestyle coach regarding the addictive nature of alcohol. I could feel myself becoming angry until it finally hit me. I was resentful of my family for modeling alcohol use at a young age and of society for normalizing and celebrating it. If I was ever going to become the person I wanted to be—the person I was meant to be—I would have to choose to live alcohol-free.

That pivotal moment ignited a profound change in my life, and I made a firm decision to never drink again—a commitment that was monumentally freeing. Saying it out loud was a breakthrough!

Ever since then, my mind has been clear, my energy has returned, along with my creativity. This decision transformed not only my health but every aspect of my life.

I instantly became more present with everyone in my life, including my wife. While it feels like a small thing, after twenty-six years of marriage, I began making the coffee every morning—a small yet significant ritual that symbolizes my renewed sense of purpose and love. I also noticed remarkable improvements in my golf and tennis games. Breaking seventy in golf was something I hadn't done in fifteen years. After becoming alcohol-free, I shot a sixty-nine at a tournament—nothing had changed except that I wasn't drinking anymore.

My work performance soared, along with my overall well-being. Out of nowhere, people began to comment that they noticed something different and how good I looked now. My body is clearly repairing and rejuvenating itself.

It has become easy to keep the weight off, my skin is clearer, my eyes are brighter, my voice is stronger, I sleep like a baby, and so much more. The changes I experienced weren't just physical or professional; they were deeply personal and spiritual. I used to pray for help with my alcohol problem during Mass. When I realized I hadn't prayed for that in six months, I just started crying. It was a prayer I'd been praying for years, and I had finally accomplished it.

Today, I feel unstoppable. My alcohol-free life has given me the energy and focus to be the best version of myself. I feel ten to fifteen years younger. My wife calls me Benjamin Button because of the changes she's seen in me. I know now that I deserve to be this person, and so does everyone I care about.

CHAPTER 6:

DEEPEN YOUR CONNECTIONS WITHOUT ALCOHOL

"First you take a drink, then the drink takes a drink, then the drink takes you."

—F. Scott Fitzgerald

D AN GO IS A CANADIAN fitness coach for entrepreneurs with one of the leading online newsletters for helping high achievers get lean, increase energy, and build a confident body. We've been friends since 2013 when we met in a business mastermind group. We see each other in person every two years at the group's meetup in Puerto Vallarta, Mexico.

Dan told me that in September 2022 he embarked on a transformative journey he called "Monk Mode," during which he decided to renounce all distractions and focus entirely on self-improvement and his business. A significant part of this journey involved giving up alcohol, a substance that had been a fixture in his life since he was eighteen years old.

Dan's relationship with alcohol began in his teenage years, sneaking drinks in his friend's basement and quickly escalated to regular partying. Throughout his twenties, Dan drank heavily, often to the point of blacking out. "Alcohol was always a part of my life. I was using alcohol as a crutch to deal with my stress and emotions."

When he stopped drinking, he was forced to face these emotions head-on, which was difficult but ultimately rewarding. "Doing hard things is actually the key to making an easier life."

Dan also experienced something of a transformation after ditching alcohol. As an introvert, he had relied on drinking to ease social anxiety. Without it, he learned to navigate social situations without needing a drink to feel comfortable. "If I need alcohol to be around a certain person or group, it's a sign that I probably don't want to be around them," he realized. This insight has allowed him to build stronger, more meaningful connections without relying on alcohol as a crutch.

Popular culture encourages you to drink, telling you that it's a way to bond with friends and family. You're passed a glass of wine to celebrate and connect. It's a key fixture at parties, dinners, dates, and work events. We think it makes us more interesting and allows us to relax.

We rarely recognize the underlying damage that drinking can cause to the very relationships we're working so hard to cultivate—but the effects to our most important connections are palpable.

One of our clients recently told us that the reason they joined *Project 90* was because they were worried about their health, early death, and missing out on time with their family. They also shared that they felt embarrassed by situations with business associates and family vacations. That's no way to live.

In this chapter, we'll explore how alcohol impacts your closest relationships and how you can navigate the conversations around your decision to quit drinking with those you care about most.

ALCOHOL'S EFFECT ON YOUR LOVE LIFE

The stats on how alcohol affects marriage and romantic relationships are quite disturbing. A recent American Addiction Centers study revealed that one in five romantic relationships cited alcohol as a factor in the decision to break up—and a quarter of couples admitted they argued when drinking. More than 22 percent of people admitted they had lied to their partner about how much they drink.[92] This study underscores the double-edged sword alcohol creates in relationship dynamics. Though drinking seems to bring people closer, it can eventually tear them apart.

Researchers have found that alcohol use disrupts intimacy in the following ways:

It makes you more irritable and aggressive: A study published in *Psychological Bulletin* found that alcohol consumption is associated with increased aggression and irritability, particularly in intimate relationships. This can escalate conflicts and lead to emotional outbursts that strain the relationship.[93]

It reduces your empathy and listening skills: Alcohol consumption can impair cognitive functions necessary for effective communication, such as empathy and listening. This often leads to misunderstandings and an inability to resolve conflicts. Research published in the *Journal of Studies on Alcohol and Drugs* highlights that alcohol impairs social cognition, making it harder for individuals to pick up on nonverbal cues or understand their partner's emotional state.[94]

It diminishes the overall quality of your relationship: Studies indicate that relationships where one or both partners frequently misuse alcohol experience lower relationship satisfaction. The American Psychological Association found that alcohol use disorders correlate with higher rates of divorce and relationship dissatisfaction. This is attributed to the stress and emotional disconnect that alcohol-related issues introduce into the relationship.[95]

If you or your partner are drinking heavily over an extended period of time, a ticking time bomb is being created—and when it blows, the consequences can range from neglecting important work or home responsibilities, to financial strain, to the potential for domestic violence.[96] One study found that 30 percent to 40 percent of the men and 27 percent to 34 percent of the women who perpetrated violence against their partners were drinking at the time of the event.[97] Furthermore, relationships affected by alcohol use disorder (AUD) show higher rates of infidelity and emotional distance, which contribute to relationship breakdowns.

Alcohol is so damaging to our relationships because it creates anxiety and irritability. At first, alcohol seems to relax us and put us in a positive mood. It's portrayed in media and culture as the key to fun, socializing, and even romance. In reality, alcohol lowers our mood and inhibitions, creating a recipe for "faster-to-fight" situations between partners.

In a 9-year study of 634 U.S. couples, marriages where one spouse was a heavy drinker had nearly a 50% divorce rate, compared to about 30% for couples where neither spouse drank heavily (see graph below) .

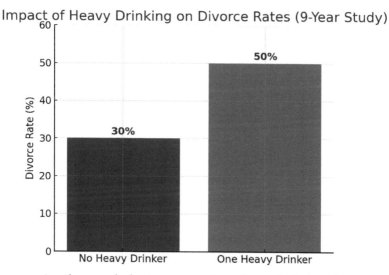

Impact of Heavy Drinking on Divorce Rates (9-Year Study)

In other words, having one partner abuse alcohol made divorce about 2x more likely.

The "alcohol myopia" theory suggests that alcohol narrows an individual's focus to immediate cues while ignoring broader situational context. This means that when someone is under the influence, they may react impulsively to immediate provocations without considering long-term consequences or other factors that would typically moderate their response.[98] Mood swings and lowered decision-making abilities can lead to increased conflicts and misunderstandings, eroding the trust and respect needed for a healthy relationship. Turns out booze is just as toxic to your marriage as it is to your body.

Many people I've worked with in our coaching programs have experienced the transformational effect cutting alcohol has had on their love life. One client, Casey, is a commercial real estate lender who quit drinking with my help. He shared that his wife had nothing but positive feedback for him once he became alcohol-free.

For my wife and me, it's huge. She sees that I think more clearly, she has seen my anxiety drop. I was only 30 days into your program and she just looked at me and said, "I've got to tell you I haven't experienced you like this since we started dating. You're just so calm." And I'm thinking, "I'm always calm, what are you talking about?" Now that's a bit of the oblivion when you have alcohol in your life.

Sometimes, all it takes is a small insight into what life is like without alcohol to understand how it's been silently sabotaging your connections and communication with others.

Blake Mycoskie is the founder of Toms Shoes and a philanthropist. In an interview on *The Ed Mylett Show*, he revealed that a thirty-day alcohol-free challenge led to his decision to consciously uncouple from his wife after seven years together.[99]

This was a small little thing... giving up two beers a night is not that big a deal... but in that, I was able to see that I really was unhappy and she was unhappy and we needed to address this.

He had previously felt obligated to stay in the relationship because of his commitment to being a great dad. So, he'd gotten into the habit of drinking a few beers or a glass of wine every night to numb himself. He decided to try thirty days alcohol-free and see how he felt. Within the first month, it was as if a fog had been lifted off his life. Mycoskie says he never would have been able to face ending his marriage without that thirty-day alcohol-free challenge.

Now, Blake says, he and his ex-wife are best friends and incredible co-parents. It makes you wonder what big important changes you could make once you stop using alcohol as a crutch and, instead, lean into life.

Some years ago, I attracted my dream partner. Does she drink? Nope. Nada. It's just never been something she's been particularly interested in. Like attracts like. Call it the Law of Attraction, but when you are health-conscious and growth-minded, you attract other health-conscious and growth-minded people.

Your intimate relationship is built on mutual respect, clear communication, and shared values. Even in happy relationships, there will be misunderstanding and conflict. However, the best thing you can do to help it thrive is to remove the potential for unnecessary conflict. Without alcohol, there are no misunderstandings blurred by intoxication and no conflicts fueled by lowered inhibitions. We are more easily able to connect on a deeper level, fully present with each other.

Be aware that even though quitting alcohol is a huge win that has the potential to improve your relationships, it's not a guarantee or a quick fix. You'll still have to do the work. That could mean attending couples counseling, working on communication skills, or resolving past conflicts.

The absence of alcohol helps us build a solid foundation based on authenticity and genuine connection. It is a reminder that when we remove substances that hinder our true selves, we can foster relationships that are enriching and fulfilling.

One *Project 90* member shared their struggles with frequently drinking to blackout and admitted they feared losing their marriage and self-respect. Their ultimate goal was to rebuild trust, portray confidence, and find peace in their daily life. If that sounds like you, you're not alone.

CONVERSATION STARTERS FOR YOUR LOVE LIFE

Building a deeper connection with your significant other can be transformative when alcohol is removed from the equation. Below are some sample conversation starters you can use to help navigate your new lifestyle with your partner and enrich your relationship. I've also included potential responses from your partner as an example.

Obviously, these are just suggestions and may not mirror real life. Use words that sound natural to you and don't expect the conversation to stop with what's on the page. These are meant to open up dialogue, not shut it down.

1. SHARING YOUR DECISION TO STOP DRINKING

Scenario: You want to share your decision to stop drinking with your partner and explain your reasons.

- » **You:** "*Hey, I've been reflecting on how alcohol fits into my life, and I'm ready to make some changes. I want to be more present and really enjoy life—and our relationship—without relying on it. I'd love your support as I go through this. How do you feel about it?*"
- » **Partner (supportive):** "*I'm behind you 100 percent. If this is important to you, I'll support it however I can.*"
- » **Partner (concerned):** "*I'm worried this will change things between us. Are we still going to enjoy nights out like we used to?*"
- » **You (response):** "*I get it. This isn't about giving up fun but finding new ways to enjoy life together. I'm also not saying I'll never have a drink again. I just think we can find new ways to connect that don't revolve around alcohol. Is this something you'd be willing to support me with?*"

Tip: Acknowledge your partner's feelings and invite them to join you in exploring new ways to enjoy time together.

2. YOUR PARTNER SHARES CONCERNS ABOUT YOUR DECISION

Scenario: Your partner is worried about the impact of your decision on your shared lifestyle.

» **Partner:** "*It feels like things won't be the same without our weekend drinks. Will I need to stop drinking too?*"

» **You:** "*I definitely understand. I'm not asking you to stop drinking, and I'm not trying to change who we are together. I'm doing this for myself, but I believe it will also strengthen our relationship. Let's take it slow and see what works for both of us.*"

Tip: Validate their concerns and reassure them that this decision is personal. Invite them to be part of your journey by suggesting activities that aren't centered on drinking.

3. DEEPENING EMOTIONAL INTIMACY WITHOUT ALCOHOL

Scenario: You want to discuss how to foster emotional closeness in your relationship without alcohol.

» **You:** "*I've realized that sometimes I've used alcohol as a crutch during tough conversations. I want to be more open and connect with you on a deeper level. How can we create moments to talk about what's truly going on?*"

» **Partner:** "*What do you mean?*"

» **You:** "*There have been times where I was nervous/ scared/anxious to talk about [insert issue] with you and I used alcohol to bury my feelings. I'd like to stop doing that so that I can connect with you in a more genuine way.*"

» **Partner:** "*How would that work?*"

» **You:** "*Maybe a simple first step we could take is to set aside a time each week to catch up about how things are going in our lives and talk about anything that's bothering us.*"

Tip: Focus on framing the conversation as a step towards more meaningful connection. Make it clear that the goal is to enhance the relationship, not just change a habit.

4. HANDLING SOCIAL EVENTS TOGETHER

Scenario: Planning how to navigate social situations without alcohol.

» **You:** *"With that dinner party coming up, I'd love to talk about how we can both enjoy ourselves without me feeling like I need to drink. It's really important to me. What do you think would work for us?"*

» **Partner (supportive):** *"Ok, great. Let's bring our own sparkling water or non-alcoholic drinks so we don't feel tempted. We could make it fun by finding some interesting mocktail recipes."*

» **Partner (hesitant):** *"I'm not sure. Won't it be awkward if everyone else is drinking and we're not?"*

» **You (response):** *"Let's keep things flexible and fun. If you want to have a drink, that's totally fine. I'm just looking for ways to feel comfortable as I work on building some new habits. Plus, now you have a built-in designated driver."*

Tip: Approach the topic collaboratively by involving your partner in the planning. Emphasize enjoying the event together rather than focusing on the absence of alcohol.

5. CULTIVATING NEW TRADITIONS TOGETHER

Scenario: Discussing new activities or rituals to strengthen your bond without alcohol.

» **You:** *"Since I'm cutting back on drinking, why don't we come up with some new activities we can enjoy together? Maybe* *we could start a tradition of exploring new hiking trails or cooking a different cuisine each month. Do you have any fun ideas that we haven't tried yet?"*

» **Partner:** *"That sounds awesome. Let's find things we're both excited about—maybe even take a class together."*

Tip: Make it about adding new, exciting experiences rather than taking something away. Involve your partner in brainstorming new traditions to make the transition more enjoyable and collaborative.

✳✳✳

Wouldn't it be great if all the difficult conversations in your life were so tidy? Reality is rarely so cut and dry. You'll have to tailor these conversations based on your personality and that of your partner. I'd even recommend you rehearse them in your head before having them. If your partner is more reserved, you might start with smaller, less direct discussions. It might take more than one conversation for you to express yourself, show that you're serious about making a change and answer their questions. For more open partners, you can dive right into deeper conversations about mutual goals.

There will certainly be some instances where your partner is resistant or downright unsupportive of your decision to stop drinking. If your partner is resistant, acknowledge their feelings without judgment. You can say something like, *"I get that this might feel like a big change, and I want you to know that my decision isn't a reflection of our relationship. I'm not asking you to change, I'm hoping that by improving myself, it'll improve our bond. This can be a positive change for both of us."*

Even so, the change to your relationship dynamic and shared experiences might be difficult. The beginning phase of your new alcohol-free life may feel strange to a partner who has only known you to be a drinker—especially if they still plan on enjoying alcohol. They may feel judged, left out, confused, or even angry with you.

Realize that if these feelings come up for them, it's not about you. Your decision is triggering something in them that is coming to the surface. The conflict that arises could actually be a good thing if you're able to talk about it openly and resolve it over time. Ultimately, the best thing you can do is to lead by example. You might be surprised to find your partner following in your footsteps if you lead the way. However, do not place expectations on them to change in any specific timeframe. Make this change for yourself without any expectations and let the rest unfold.

ALCOHOL'S EFFECT ON YOUR PARENT-CHILD RELATIONSHIP

Our clients have shared some of their deepest regrets around alcohol, and overwhelmingly those regrets revolve around how drinking affected their relationships with their children. For many parents struggling with Alcohol Use Disorder (AUD), it's part of a cycle handed down through generations. Some of us are simply repeating the same coping mechanisms that we watched our parents use. We might think that one or two drinks are harmless, but, in reality, even "casual" alcohol use can subtly but powerfully alter the way we show up for our kids. Many of the clients we work with struggle with much more than casual drinking, too.

One *Project 90* participant admitted that their cycles of binge drinking made them "feel trapped and exhausted," leaving them unfocused and unable to be present for their children. Their reason for quitting alcohol was to foster healthier relationships with their family and live regret-free.

Another member opened up about their struggle, saying, "My drinking spiraled after my divorce. It's my way to cope with stress, especially with my daughter's attitude. I drink to pass the time, but it's ruining my sleep, energy, and confidence." Your kids notice these things.

Children, regardless of their age, are extremely perceptive. They see changes in a parent's behavior, mood, and presence, even when we think we're hiding it well. These shifts can create confusion, fear, and even resentment toward the parent. They begin to associate alcohol with unpredictable moods, inconsistency, or even outright absence, and these associations can follow them well into adulthood. The impact of alcohol abuse on your children may not always be visible, but over time, it can become a significant barrier to genuine connection.

Here are some of the most significant ways drinking can impact your relationship with your children.

Reduced Emotional Availability

One of the first ways alcohol impacts the parent-child relationship is by diminishing emotional availability. When under the influence, it's more challenging to be fully present. Alcohol impairs a parent's ability to respond to their child's needs consistently, which leads to emotional disconnect. This absence is particularly damaging because children, especially when they're young, look to their parents for validation, guidance, and comfort. They need to know that they have a reliable source of love and stability, yet alcohol clouds that consistency.

Consider a scenario where your child is excitedly sharing something with you—an achievement at school, a personal milestone, or even a problem they're struggling with. When alcohol is involved, reactions may vary from lukewarm engagement to irritation or dismissal. Without realizing it, parents can leave their children feeling invalidated or even burdensome, pushing them to seek emotional support elsewhere or suppress their feelings altogether. Over time, this pattern erodes the trust and security that should define the parent-child bond.

Lowered Impulse Control and Increased Aggression

Alcohol lowers inhibitions and increases irritability, which can make even the calmest parents react unpredictably. When children experience their parents' alcohol-induced anger or frustration, it can be frightening and confusing, especially if they're too young to understand why it's happening. Something as minor as a messy room or a sibling argument might escalate into a shouting match or even a physical confrontation. These experiences create an environment of fear and unpredictability, leaving children on edge, unsure of how their parent will respond at any given moment.

Over time, these heightened reactions can have lasting psychological effects. Children might start "walking on eggshells" around the parent, becoming overly cautious or even emotionally withdrawn to avoid triggering an outburst. The lack of impulse control associated with alcohol use can thus lead to a family dynamic characterized by tension and unspoken resentment. Eventually, this tension undermines the parent's authority and can lead to deeper emotional rifts within the family.

Diminished Trust and Safety

Trust is foundational to any healthy relationship, and for children, feeling safe and trusting in their parents is paramount. When a parent's behavior becomes erratic or inconsistent because of alcohol, it shakes the child's sense of stability and safety. For example, promises made while sober can easily be forgotten or dismissed under the influence, whether it's attending an event, helping with homework, or simply being there for a conversation. This inconsistency leads to disappointment and can make children feel unimportant or even abandoned.

As these experiences accumulate, children might start distancing themselves emotionally. They may develop a self-protective habit of keeping their feelings or concerns to themselves, wary of relying on a parent who might let them down. This erosion of trust is a gradual process, but it can be incredibly difficult to rebuild once damaged, especially as children grow older and form lasting impressions of their parent's reliability.

Modeling of Unhealthy Coping Mechanisms

Perhaps one of the most significant and often overlooked impacts of alcohol use is the example it sets for children on how to handle life's challenges. Parents are the primary role models for their children, and kids often internalize their behaviors, including how they cope with stress, sadness, and conflict. When alcohol is a go-to mechanism for managing emotions, children may come to see it as a normal or even necessary way to cope. This creates a dangerous cycle, increasing their likelihood of turning to substances when faced with their own hardships.

Many children of parents with AUD are statistically more likely to struggle with substance use disorders themselves, as they replicate the patterns they observed growing up. In trying to handle life's pressures, they fall back on what they've learned: that alcohol is a means of escape or comfort. This inherited coping strategy not only affects their own lives but can carry into future generations if not addressed. Breaking this cycle is a powerful motivation for parents to consider how their choices affect not just their own well-being but also the lives and futures of their children.

PRACTICAL CONVERSATION STARTERS FOR BUILDING AN ALCOHOL-FREE CONNECTION WITH YOUR CHILDREN

Opening up a conversation about alcohol with your children, no matter their age, is a powerful step toward rebuilding trust and showing them a healthier way forward. These dialogues don't have to be perfect. They likely won't be much like the simple scripts we've written below. It's ok if they're scary. There may even be tears.

They just need to be honest.

Each of these conversation starters is a way to open up, listen, and let your children express themselves, whether they're young kids, teenagers, or adults. These conversations can be the beginning of a new chapter, where you model healthy coping mechanisms and emotional availability.

FOR YOUNG CHILDREN

Young children thrive on routine, reliability, and reassurance. They lack the cognitive maturity to understand why their parent might be acting differently, so they often blame themselves for the shifts they observe. This confusion can lead to anxiety, attachment issues, and emotional dysregulation as they struggle to reconcile the "two versions" of their parent: the one who is present and engaged and the one altered by alcohol.

Here's how you can open up a conversation with your young child:

1. Explaining Why You're Making Changes

First, you'll want to explain to a young child why you're no longer drinking.

> » **You:** "*You might notice that I'm not drinking the way I used to. I've decided to stop because I want to be the best parent I can be for you, and I realized that drinking was making that harder. This way, I can spend even more time having fun with you and be there whenever you need me.*"
> » **Child's Potential Response:** "*Will you still be the same?*"
> » **You:** "*Absolutely! I'll still be the same me, but this change will actually make me even more 'me.' I'll be able to focus better, be there for you even more, and spend time doing things we both love.*"

2. Encouraging Their Open Feelings

Next, invite your young child to share how they're feeling and gently address any confusion.

> » **You:** "*Sometimes I might not have been as patient or as fun as I could have been because of drinking. I want to make sure you feel good about talking to me if something makes you feel sad or confused. If there's anything you're worried about, I'd love to hear it so we can work on it together.*"
> » **Child's Potential Response:** "*Sometimes I felt like you were mad at me.*"
> » **You:** "*I'm really sorry if I ever made you feel that way. I want to make sure you feel safe and happy with me. Thank you for telling me, and please know that you can always talk to me about anything that's on your mind.*"

FOR ADOLESCENTS

Teenagers are navigating a complex developmental stage, balancing independence with a need for parental support. When a parent struggles with alcohol, teens may feel embarrassed, resentful, or even hostile, especially if drinking has caused them to miss out on support during critical moments. Adolescents may act out, use substances themselves, or become distant, as they struggle with conflicting emotions about their parent's behavior.

Here's how you can open up a conversation with your teen about your drinking:

1. Acknowledging the Impact of Your Drinking

First, you'll want to acknowledge how your drinking may have affected your relationship with your teenager.

> » **You:** "*I know there might have been times when I wasn't fully there for you because of drinking—for instance [INSERT*

SPECIFIC EXAMPLE HERE]. *I wanted to let you know that I'm sorry for any hurt that was caused. I'm making this change because I want to be the best parent I can be for you, and I want to rebuild our relationship. How does that make you feel?"*

» **Teen's Potential Response:** *"I don't know. I've been let down before, so I'm not sure if things will really change."*

» **You:** *"I understand. It makes sense to feel that way, especially if you've felt disappointed before. I'm not expecting everything to be perfect right away, but I'm ready to show you, one step at a time, that this change is real. If there's anything specific that would help you feel supported, please let me know. I'm here to listen and to start rebuilding our trust."*

2. Opening Up About Why You're Quitting

Next, explain your "why" to a teenager and invite them into the journey.

» **You:** *"I've realized that I want to be fully there for you and support you in the best way I can. Drinking was getting in the way of that. So, I've decided to stop, and I'm really excited about the chance to reconnect with you and have a relationship that's built on more than just daily routines. I'd like us to have more fun together and build trust that lasts."*

» **Teen's Potential Response:** *"You're always going to be busy with other things."*

» **You:** *"I get it. I do have a lot on my plate, but this is important enough to me that I'm willing to make it a priority. Let's start by finding a few things we can do together each week—things you actually enjoy. It doesn't have to be anything huge; it's just about being together and building a stronger connection."*

FOR ADULT CHILDREN

Adult children are often deeply impacted by a parent's alcohol use, even if they no longer live at home. They may feel conflicted between love and resentment, especially if alcohol has caused ongoing issues in the family. Adult children may cope by creating emotional or physical distance, or they may feel compelled to "fix" or enable their parent, leading to codependency. These relationships can be challenging to navigate, but healing is possible with honest communication and support.

Here's how to open up a conversation with your adult children:

1. Acknowledging Past Issues You've Caused

First, you'll want to open the door to discuss past hurts with your adult child, acknowledging the impact of your past actions.

- » **You:** *"I know there were times when my drinking may have caused pain or disappointment. I'm sorry for that, and I know it can't be undone. But I'd like to talk about it and hear how you're feeling about our relationship. If there's anything you want to share or anything I can do to support you, I'm here."*
- » **Adult Child's Potential Response:** *"It's hard to just move on from everything that happened. I don't know if talking about it will really help."*
- » **You:** *"I completely understand. I don't expect us to just move past things quickly or to pretend it was easy. But I want you to know that I'm here, and I'm ready to listen whenever you feel comfortable. I'm committed to making things better, step by step, and that means being present for you and showing up as the best version of myself."*

2. Reassuring Your Commitment to Change

Next, offer reassurance to your adult child that you're committed to lasting change and expressing your intentions.

» **You:** "*I realize it might be difficult to trust that this change will really stick, especially since I've disappointed you before. I want you to know that I'm committed to this change, and I'm doing it for myself and for us, so we can have the kind of relationship we both deserve. I'm here to be a more present, reliable parent for you now.*"

» **Adult Child's Potential Response:** "*That's good to hear. I'm just skeptical because you've said similar things before.*"

» **You:** "*You're right, and I understand why you'd feel that way. This time, I'm not just talking about change—I'm putting in the work. It's not something I expect you to believe overnight, but I'm ready to show you, through actions and consistency, that I'm serious. This is about building a new foundation for our relationship that we can both feel good about.*"

These conversations most likely will not be "clean"—they may come with a lot of tough moments as you remember times when you did not show up as your best self for the people you love most. Do not despair. Mark these moments as the beginning of a powerful healing shift in your relationship with your children. They're not about perfection or immediate results but about showing up honestly and giving them the reassurance they deserve. Each conversation offers a chance to rebuild trust, address the past, and create a healthier, alcohol-free future together.

ALCOHOL'S EFFECT ON YOUR FRIENDSHIPS

Your friendships, professional relationships, and wider community will all experience significant upgrades when you quit drinking, too. One of the more unexpected things that happened when I quit alcohol was an upgrade in my social circle. I went from spending time with friends at bars to having deeper conversations with new friends in gyms, farmers markets, and growth-minded seminars and workshops.

To be clear, there wasn't anything inherently wrong with my existing relationships, but I discovered that I started attracting a different kind of person, those with a more open-minded and positive mindset, almost immediately after quitting.

We tend to be influenced by the people we spend the most time with. When I decided to go alcohol-free, I didn't consciously sever ties with all my friends who weren't. They were still my friends, and many remain so. I did, however, notice that I naturally spent more time with those who drank only moderately or not at all. The relationships in my life became so much more energizing and fulfilling.

When I did catch up with my heavy-drinking friends, most would give me a hard time about my lifestyle choice. They would tease me, make light of my decision, and sometimes even try to persuade me to have "just one drink." However, my new friends either encouraged me to stay on the path of the alcohol-free journey or, quite frankly, didn't care at all. It simply wasn't an issue and was rarely a discussion.

This natural shift toward spending more time with those who favor moderate or no drinking didn't feel like a loss. Instead, it felt like a gain. The relationships that I formed were more energizing and fulfilling. Each interaction felt more genuine, and the connections I made were deeper and more meaningful.

One profound shift I noticed after quitting alcohol was my focus on contributing to others. Nobel Peace Prize winner Aung San Suu Kyi's words in *Freedom from Fear*[100] resonated with me: "If you're feeling helpless, help someone." Cutting alcohol out of my life made room for me to think more about how I could support and uplift my friends rather than how they could support me.

This focus on others has directly benefitted me in my personal life. Several years ago, I read Keith Ferrazzi's book *Never Eat Alone*, and it completely changed how I see relationships. In the book, Keith suggests that instead of asking how others can help you, you should become curious about how you can help them. I began to take this approach and ironically, I now end up getting a lot more help because of it. It's funny how that works.

I got creative with events and entertainment—meeting friends and clients for biking, yoga, cultural events, and hikes. It was no longer about meeting up at a bar to drink but about engaging in activities that promote well-being and connection. I found that people enjoyed doing something new and different, not just sitting at the bar.

These new approaches to socializing not only enhanced my relationships but also broadened my social horizons. I became more involved in my community and built stronger bonds with those around me. The joy of helping others became a powerful motivator for maintaining my alcohol-free lifestyle.

CONVERSATION STARTERS FOR YOUR FRIENDSHIPS

Navigating friendships while embracing an alcohol-free lifestyle can present unique challenges. These sample dialogues and scripts will help you articulate your choice and foster deeper connections with friends, demonstrating that fun and meaningful relationships don't require alcohol.

1. Explaining Your Decision to Be Alcohol-Free

Scenario: You're out with friends, and they notice you're not drinking.

> » **Friend:** *"Hey, why aren't you drinking tonight?"*
> » **You:** *"I've decided to take a break from alcohol for a while. I'm focusing on feeling my best and seeing what life is like without it. Plus, I'm still here to enjoy the night with you all—just minus the drinks"*

Tip: Keep the tone light and focus on the positive reasons behind your decision. Share how it's a personal choice rather than a judgment on anyone else's habits.

2. Reassuring Your Friends That You're Still Fun

Scenario: Your friends are worried that you might not enjoy going out like you used to.

> » **Friend:** *"Are you sure you won't miss out? You used to be the life of the party"*
> » **You:** *"I get where you're coming from, but honestly, I feel like I'm enjoying our time even more now. I'm still the same person, just without the next-day regrets. Trust me, I'll keep bringing the good vibes"*

Tip: Emphasize that you're still fully present and engaged. Reassuring them that you're not missing out and can still have fun helps shift their perspective.

3. Suggesting Alcohol-Free Alternatives

Scenario: Your friends suggest meeting at a bar, but you'd prefer a different type of outing.

> » **You:** *"Hey, we've been hitting the same bars for ages. How about we mix things up? There's a cool escape room nearby or we could try out that new night market. It might be fun to do something different"*

Tip: Frame the suggestion as a chance to explore new activities rather than avoiding bars. This shifts the focus from alcohol to the shared experience of trying something novel.

4. Handling Teasing Lightheartedly

Scenario: Your friends tease you about not drinking.
> » **Friend:** *"Don't be a buzzkill. Just have one drink."*
> » **You:** *"I'm just here to make sure you all have a designated hype person. Besides, who's going to remember all the ridiculous things you say if I don't keep my head clear?"*

Tip: Keep the response playful and use humor to defuse the situation. It shows that you're confident in your decision while still engaging with the group's dynamic.

5. Openly Discussing Social Anxiety

Scenario: A friend asks if you're not drinking because you're anxious.

> » **Friend:** "*So, you're not drinking because it makes you anxious?*"
> » **You:** "*Actually, I realized I was using alcohol to manage my anxiety, but now I'm challenging myself to be more present without it. It's been a good change, and I'm finding I can relax and have fun without needing a drink.*"

Tip: Be honest without going into too much detail. Sharing a little about your personal growth can open up a deeper conversation if your friend is curious, but it also keeps the discussion light if they're just making casual conversation.

Similar to your romantic relationship, learn to read the room when it comes to declaring your intention to quit drinking. For instance, if you're with a group of close friends, you can be more candid about why you're making such a big change. For newer friends or acquaintances, keep explanations shorter and emphasize the fun aspects of staying alcohol-free. This is not a death sentence.

It's also important to remember that while quitting alcohol can certainly enhance clarity and communication in your friendships, the recipe for a good relationship is far more complex than just removing alcohol. Factors like personality differences, emotional compatibility, and communication styles also play major roles in the success of your relationships—so if you find yourself drifting away from friends because you're no longer drinking with them, it's a good sign that something is missing.

With your newfound clarity, you can choose to improve the relationship or let it go. If a friend seems resistant or uncomfortable with your decision to quit, you could say something like, *"I'm just trying this out for a bit. It doesn't mean I'm not here to enjoy the night. Let's just see how it goes."*

ALCOHOL'S EFFECT ON YOUR PROFESSIONAL RELATIONSHIPS

The choice to forgo drinking used to be an anomaly in the business world. Increasingly, it's becoming the norm. Leaders, entrepreneurs, and high performers are awakening to quitting drinking as a key to unlocking peak performance. Millions of Americans are increasingly choosing the alcohol-free lifestyle as a strategy for success.

Indeed, some of the world's most successful investors, entrepreneurs, artists, and celebrities credit much of their success to their decision to live alcohol-free. These high achievers include billionaires like Berkshire Hathaway chairman Warren Buffett, Oracle founder Larry Elisson, and *Huffington Post* founder Arianna Huffington, to name a few.

Buffett says he has never drunk alcohol, amassing a $60 billion fortune in the process.

"It's the weakest link that causes the problem," Buffett once said. "Alcohol is a real 'weakest link' problem." Buffett's friend and Berkshire Hathaway vice chairman, the late Charlie Munger, also didn't drink. He's been quoted as saying,[101]

"The four closest friends of my youth were highly intelligent, ethical, humorous types, favored in person and background. Two are long dead, with alcohol a contributing factor, and a third is a living alcoholic, if you call that living. I have yet to meet anyone, in over six decades of life, whose

life was worsened by over fear and over avoidance of such a deceptive pathway to destruction."

Oracle founder Larry Ellison told biographer Matthew Symonds that he "can't stand" anything that clouds his mind. "I have no problem with people drinking," he said. "If that's what they want to do, God bless them, that's their business. But I can't do those things."[102]

Silicon Valley is taking note, with tech companies reevaluating their alcohol policies. The culture of binge drinking is well-known among tech startups, with their fridges full of free beer and regular happy hours to help employees relax and stay engaged. In fact, one survey found that tech is the number-one industry that allows or sponsors alcohol consumption. It's worth noting that more than half of the employees from tech companies like Microsoft, Amazon, Google, Uber, and Facebook report experiencing symptoms of burnout.

"It's such a part of the culture, especially here in San Francisco, that I would go out for dinner and have two to three drinks every day," Silicon Valley entrepreneur Justin Kan, the CEO of law-tech startup Atrium, recently told CNN. He noted, however, that he had recently seen a shift within his tech circle. "I was at a dinner with a lot of tech people last night and probably half the people weren't drinking."[103]

As we discussed earlier, alcohol hurts productivity and performance, which impacts your ability to reach your potential at work—and your bottom line. Removing it creates space for clear communication, mutual respect, and genuine support. However, you may be hesitant to stop drinking if everybody else is. Here are some conversation starters to help you navigate quitting alcohol in your professional circle.

1. Addressing Alcohol at Work Events

Scenario: At a work event where alcohol is available, colleagues notice you're not drinking.

- » **Coworker:** "Hey You're not drinking? What's up with that?"
- » **You:** "I'm trying out an alcohol-free lifestyle to keep my energy up and stay sharp. I'm here to enjoy the company and the conversation—no drinks needed." .

Tip: Keep the focus on the positive benefits and emphasize that you're still fully engaged in the social aspect.

2. Responding to Curiosity About Your Choice

Scenario: A colleague wonders why you're not joining the usual after-work drinks.

- » **Colleague:** "Why aren't you joining us for drinks after work?"
- » **You:** "I'm focusing on personal goals and finding that I'm more productive without alcohol. It's been a game-changer for my clarity and motivation."

Tip: Frame your choice as a part of personal development, making it clear that it's about growth rather than judgment of others' choices.

3. Handling a Drunken Coworker Lightheartedly

Scenario: A coworker playfully tries to persuade you to have a drink.

- » **Coworker:** "Come on, just one drink with us."
- » **You:** "Thanks, but I'm sticking to my health goals. I'll still be the life of the party—I'm just doing it with my sparkling water."

Tip: Use humor to lighten the situation and show that you're still participating without compromising your choice.

4. Politely Declining Invitations to Drink

Scenario: A colleague insists you join the after-work drinks, and you want to decline gracefully.

> » **Colleague:** *"You have to join us. It'll be fun."*
> » **You:** *"I appreciate the invite, but I'm skipping drinks for now. I've been feeling so good without alcohol, and I'm motivated to keep it up. Let's catch up at lunch one day instead."*

Tip: Offer an alternative to show you're still interested in connecting, just in a different setting.

5. Discussing the Benefits of Your Decision

Scenario: Colleagues discuss how they're feeling sluggish from the weekend's drinking, and you want to share your experience.

> » **You:** *"I used to feel the same way, but since I cut out alcohol, I've noticed a big difference in my energy levels and focus. It's amazing how much clearer my mind feels."*

Tip: Share your experience as an anecdote rather than advice, making it clear that it's your personal journey.

6. Clarifying Your Personal Boundaries During a Work Event

Scenario: You need to assert your decision when coworkers pressure you during an office party.

> » **Coworker:** *"Just one drink won't hurt, right?"*
> » **You:** *"I appreciate the thought, but I'm really committed to staying alcohol-free. I'm here to enjoy the event, and I'm having a great time as is."*

Tip: Set boundaries respectfully, and reaffirm that you're fully present at the event without needing alcohol.

7. Explaining Your New Lifestyle to Supportive Coworkers
Scenario: A coworker asks about your choice to live alcohol-free.

> » **Colleague:** *"I noticed that you're not drinking. What made you decide to quit?"*
> » **You:** *"I realized alcohol was holding me back from reaching my full potential, both at work and personally. Now I feel more energized and focused, and it's motivating me to keep growing."*

Tip: Emphasize the positive changes and how they're impacting your professional life to help your colleague understand the full context.

✳✳✳

Every work culture is different. In some workplaces, it may be better to keep explanations brief, focusing on health or personal preferences. In more open environments, sharing a bit about your motivations can foster deeper connections. Remember, you don't owe anybody an explanation. If a coworker is persistent, you can say, *"I'm just trying it out for a bit. It doesn't mean I won't ever join in again, but right now I'm enjoying the benefits."*

With your romantic, platonic and professional relationships, you'll likely see a significant improvement in the quality of communication and overall satisfaction once you quit drinking. And the best part is, embracing an alcohol-free lifestyle not only benefits your own well-being but can also inspire a shift in those around you. Just wait until you witness the positive ripple effect of your decision.

Of course, the most important relationship is the one you have with yourself. In the next chapter, we'll look at how quitting alcohol can be a gateway to sustainable joy and I'll provide specific tools to help facilitate long-term fulfillment in your life.

Ready to begin your journey to becoming alcohol-free?
Get tools, support, and free resources at
www.alcoholfreelifestyle.com/resources

KEY TAKEAWAYS

» True connections don't need alcohol—relationships deepen when built on clear communication and genuine presence.

» Removing alcohol can strengthen your love life, reducing conflict and creating healthier, more stable relationships.

» Friendships thrive without alcohol, attracting positive, like-minded people and more meaningful social experiences.

» Sobriety enhances professional relationships, boosting clarity, energy, and leadership in your career.

CHAPTER 6 REFLECTION POINTS

Write out the answers to the following prompts in your favorite journal to create simple, concrete action steps for your alcohol-free journey.

Reflection: How has alcohol affected my ability to show up fully and authentically in my relationships?

Question: What fears do I have about socializing or connecting without alcohol, and are they truly valid?

Next Step: What is one way I can practice building deeper, more meaningful connections without the influence of alcohol?

"I STRENGTHENED MY MARRIAGE AND SAVED 5 MILLION HEARTBEATS THIS YEAR"

By Evan Melcher
Financial Adviser
Alpharetta, Georgia

I N 2021, I DECIDED TO take a ninety-day break from alcohol so that I could be fully focused on my family and serving my clients. As a numbers guy, I have always been very interested in data. I have been wearing both an Apple Watch and Oura Ring for several years now, and I closely track my health metrics.

I decided to see if my ninety-day hiatus from alcohol would allow me to taper

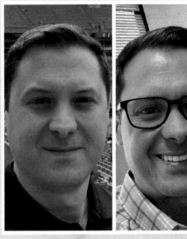

Evan is happier and healthier than ever living alcohol-free.

my reliance on some of the medications I was taking after a back surgery. Frankly, my doctors and I have been blown away by the results and I am proud to report that I am no longer taking ANY prescription medication.

My cholesterol, which was considered to be "elevated" or "high" is now normal without the use of statins. The acid reflux, which kept me awake at night and led to several endoscopies and daily medication, is now under control without medication. Finally, I was able to stop my anti-anxiety medications as I have felt more even, centered, and balanced in the past year.

As I have tracked my health over the past year, I have also seen other significant benefits. First of all, my sleep has dramatically improved. The Oura Ring assigns a Sleep Score based on the quality of your sleep each night. When I was drinking wine at night, my Sleep Score would regularly be in the 70s or low 80s, indicating suboptimal sleep quality and fewer hours of deep restorative sleep. In the past year, my Sleep Score has been in the high 80s and even low 90s, indicating that I am now getting higher quality, more restorative sleep to help me function more optimally during my waking hours.

Another health benefit I've seen is the impact on my resting heart rate. Since going alcohol-free a year ago, my resting heart rate has fallen by over ten beats per minute. Are you kidding me? That's over 5 million heartbeats per year.

Other than the aforementioned health benefits, the most profound upgrade I have experienced is the quality of my family interactions. I have an amazing wife and two beautiful children at home. Going alcohol-free has coincided with richer experiences with my family, and I feel like I have more patience and am more engaged in life's daily experiences. As I look to the future, I am so fired up about the opportunity to be fully present and invested in each experience.

Now that I have gone years without alcohol, you might wonder what's next. Forever is a long time, so I won't make any promises... but at this time I don't feel a burning desire to get off this train. I plan to continue working on and investing in myself so that I can show up fully for my family, friends, clients, and community. I truly appreciate those that have helped me on this journey, and I look forward to the future.

PART III:

BEGINNING YOUR ALCOHOL-FREE LIFESTYLE

CHAPTER 7:

CULTIVATING SUSTAINABLE JOY

"Alcohol is the reduced form of Spirit. Therefore, many people, lacking Spirit, take to drink. They fill themselves with alcohol."

—CARL JUNG

I N HIS 1951 CLASSIC THE *Wisdom of Insecurity*, renowned philosopher Alan Watts made a very poignant observation about those struggling with alcohol use disorder:

> *One of the world's most vicious circles is the problem of the alcoholic. In very many cases he knows quite clearly that he is destroying himself, that, for him, liquor is poison, that he actually hates being drunk, and even dislikes the taste of liquor. For, dislike it as he may, the experience of not drinking is worse. It gives him the "horrors," because he stands face to face with the unveiled, basic insecurity of the world.*

It stands to reason that Watts would have such a penetrating view into the mind of someone struggling with alcohol. In a morbid twist of irony, Watts died of heart failure related to alcoholism. If, as Watts suggests, alcohol is a crutch used by the masses to deal with life's hardships, then removing alcohol is a pathway to dealing with fear and uncertainty standing on your own two feet.

Most busy professionals experience varying levels of stress, anxiety, and depression. It's almost impossible not to get overwhelmed if you're pushing hard. Alcohol is a temporary pain reliever for mental, emotional and physical injuries. Long-term, however, it is a medicine that kills more than it cures by dulling your emotions and making it harder to experience true joy.

Clients who quit drinking regularly share updates with me as to how they're feeling. Most say things like "I love who I am," "I feel great," and "Everything feels better." They're feeling this way because as damaging toxins from alcohol are being removed from their body, their natural state of calm, clarity, and focus is free to flourish.

From this state, joy can flow.

IS ALCOHOL STOPPING YOU FROM HEALING?

It's easy to waste decades of your life mistaking the temporary pleasure you get from drinking for true fulfillment or happiness. First, let's make a distinction between pleasure and fulfillment.

Pleasure is heavily tied to the dopamine system, which is responsible for the brain's reward pathway. When you consume alcohol, dopamine is released, creating a temporary "high" that reinforces the behavior and encourages repeated use. This surge in dopamine creates a cycle of chasing pleasure because the brain becomes conditioned to seek out the same activity that led to the dopamine release. However, the more alcohol you consume, the less effective it becomes at producing the same level of satisfaction. That's when tolerance sets in.[104]

Pleasure is all about what feels good right now. It's a happening that you experience, not a state you can maintain indefinitely. Pleasure is a sensation that comes and goes like an electrical current. Here one moment, gone the next. You cannot capture it, because the more you feed the pleasure monster, the more demanding it becomes. It's never satisfied. That's why pleasure alone is not a reliable foundation for building a meaningful, fulfilling life.

Unlike pleasure, fulfillment is connected to the brain's prefrontal cortex, which is involved in long-term planning, self-control, and the pursuit of meaningful goals. Activities that require delayed gratification, such as working toward a professional goal, exercising, or practicing mindfulness, activate and strengthen this part of the brain. These activities may not always be enjoyable in the moment but contribute to a deeper sense of satisfaction with life.[105]

Fulfillment is all about long-term, sustained happiness. It isn't worried about whether you're uncomfortable today. It's concerned with your highest vision for yourself. It feels fulfilling when you know that you're living up to your potential. Those looking for fulfillment out of life will do things that aren't fun now, to reap massive rewards later. If you're a busy, successful professional, you know all about delayed gratification.

Alcohol is particularly good at numbing short-term pain and increasing pleasure instantaneously. Push the button, get the stimulus. The stimulation dulls the anxiety and existential uncertainty of being a human in society. It feels good to feel good. So why not try to feel good all the time? The problem is that feeling good now often doesn't lead to feeling good later. Over time, with more drinking, the dopamine surge from alcohol diminishes until it's almost nonexistent. This prevents you from being able to feel joy and satisfaction from other types of experiences. Drinking alcohol puts a lid on how good you can feel when you're not drinking. It has a similar effect on you that overexposure to porn will have on your enjoyment of real sex. It makes real life duller.[106]

There's an Instagram quote I'll paraphrase, which has been massively overshared but is relevant here: "Easy life now, hard life later. Hard life now, easy life later." This quote reminds me that by embracing short-term challenges, discomfort becomes a signal of growth rather than something to avoid. Alcohol is an easy short-term solution to pain, stress, and anxiety. There's no doubt about it. The question is: How much long-term happiness are you sacrificing in exchange for short-term numbing?

Here's a paradox for you to explore: If you are experiencing pain that you constantly feel the need to numb through the use of alcohol, the numbing you're getting from the alcohol may also be the very thing stopping you from healing the pain you're experiencing. In other words: you have to feel it to heal it.

Alcohol has a profound effect on the amygdala and hippocampus—areas of the brain that process emotions and form memories.[107] Several studies have found that using alcohol to numb negative emotions interrupts the brain's ability to properly process and resolve those feelings. Over time, this avoidance can actually amplify anxiety and emotional distress, making the original problems more pronounced. Facing difficult emotions sober, though it can be excruciating, allows the brain to form new connections and coping mechanisms, which are critical for emotional resilience and healing. Booze is actually stopping you from getting to the root of whatever problem you are using it to numb or solve.

Here's another paradox to consider: healing doesn't usually feel good at first. That's because it requires addressing the root causes of your emotional pain, not just treating the symptoms. You're not looking for a painkiller. You're looking for healing and a return to your true, whole self. That means getting to know yourself better without the mask of alcohol. Healing will be found by learning to love yourself and learning to process the emotions you're feeling instead of pushing them down with another drink. Working through your emotions sober is the key to unlocking the solution to whatever your unique struggle in life is. As bestselling author Ryan Holiday would say, "The obstacle is the way."

USING THE 4S MODEL TO KILL ALCOHOL CRAVINGS

A friend of mine, Cory Muscara, is a mindfulness teacher and former monk who spent years meditating in silence, and he now teaches people how to cultivate deep presence and live more fulfilling lives through mindfulness practices. Muscara is the author of the book *Stop Missing Your Life: How to Be Deeply Present in an Un-Present World*.

In a recent conversation on my podcast, we delved into the complexities of alcohol cravings and the power of mindfulness in overcoming them. Muscara's deep insights into the human mind stem from his intensive meditation practice in Burma, where he learned to appreciate the clarity and joy of a mind free from external substances. His teachings now focus on helping people cultivate presence and live more fulfilling lives through mindfulness.

As someone who has never had a deeply complicated relationship with alcohol, Muscara's perspective is both relatable and enlightening. He shared with me that while he did drink during his college years, it was never his go-to coping mechanism. Instead, he gravitated more toward stimulants like caffeine and, at one point, even nicotine, which he mistakenly believed was beneficial for cognitive performance.

Reflecting on his past, Cory told me, "I was never someone who would go for a drink to numb or to wind down. It was always in particular contexts, like partying."

After returning from his time in Burma, where he practiced intense, daily meditation, he became highly sensitized to the effects of alcohol and other substances on his mental clarity. He described this transformation, stating, "I had just really appreciated what a clear, bright, happy mind feels like without any exogenous substances. I got really sensitized to that, and really sensitized to anything that would make that dull."

This newfound sensitivity made him less inclined to reach for alcohol, even in social settings where drinking is the norm. He explained that as he began to experience the joy of living with a clear mind, the idea of consuming alcohol became less appealing.

"I really got sensitized to the joy of clarity and being lucid and really like being in my life that made me, like, not want to mess with it even more," he shared. "I saw that I could have a great time, even if people were drinking around me. And I liked feeling good the next morning. I didn't feel like I couldn't relax or have fun without alcohol."

In addition to sharing his personal journey, Muscara also offered practical advice for dealing with alcohol cravings, which can be incredibly challenging for many people. He introduced his 4S Model, a mindfulness-based approach designed to help individuals navigate and overcome cravings.

The model consists of four steps:

1. See
2. Sympathize
3. Soften
4. Surround

The first step, **See**, involves acknowledging the craving without judgment.

"The first S is just the willingness to see it clearly, to turn toward the energy of the craving," Muscara explained. This step is crucial because it involves facing the craving head-on rather than trying to ignore or suppress it.

The second step, **Sympathize**, encourages individuals to recognize that the craving stems from a place of pain or discomfort.

"The craving itself, that place in you it's coming from, is suffering. It's in pain. It doesn't want to feel this way," Muscara said. By offering compassion to oneself during these moments, the craving is met with understanding rather than resistance.

The third step, **Soften**, focuses on relaxing the body, which often becomes tense during cravings. Muscara emphasized the importance of softening the areas where tension is most noticeable, such as the hands, belly, or chest.

"Typically, we get that release by getting the drink or the thing that we're craving. But if you actually just relax the body, soften where that area is tensioning, you get some of that release without having to fulfill the craving," he explained.

Finally, the fourth step, **Surround**, involves surrounding the craving with love and compassion. Muscara suggests imagining the craving as a hurt child that needs care and attention.

"Imagine the craving almost like you're welcoming it into your heart. You're holding it in your heart and caring for it," he said. This approach helps to dissipate the craving's power, reducing its grip on the individual.

HOW TO IMPLEMENT THE 4S MODEL INTO YOUR LIFE

Cravings will come, but luckily, now you have a tool to bring yourself back to center. Here's how you can effectively implement the 4S Model into your life when you're feeling the urge to drink.

1. See

Acknowledge the craving without judgment. The first step is to bring awareness to the craving as it arises. This involves recognizing the urge and observing it objectively, rather than suppressing or reacting impulsively to it. Techniques to help with this include:

- » **Label the craving:** Mentally identify the feeling with phrases like, "I notice the urge to drink" or "I feel a strong craving." This helps to create a mental distance between yourself and the craving.
- » **Breathe deeply:** Take a few slow, deep breaths to center yourself and anchor your awareness in the present moment. Breathing can calm the nervous system and provide clarity.
- » **Journaling:** Writing down your thoughts and feelings about the craving can help you gain insights into its triggers. Describe the situation, the intensity of the craving, and any emotions tied to it.

Example: If you experience a craving after a stressful day at work, you might say to yourself, "I'm noticing a strong urge to drink because I'm feeling overwhelmed." This simple acknowledgment can reduce the craving's power.

2. Sympathize

Recognize that the craving arises from a place of discomfort or pain. Understanding that cravings are often rooted in emotional distress can help shift your approach from resistance to compassion.

» **Use self-compassion phrases:** Practice self-talk that acknowledges your struggles kindly. For example, say, "It's okay to feel this way. I'm doing my best in a challenging situation."

» **Identify emotional triggers:** Reflect on whether the craving is linked to specific emotions, such as stress, loneliness, or boredom. Once you recognize the source, you can address the underlying need in a healthier way, such as by talking to a friend or practicing a relaxing activity.

» **Remember your humanity:** Cravings are a natural part of being human. Everyone experiences discomfort and has coping mechanisms. Remind yourself that you're not alone in this struggle.

Example: When feeling lonely, acknowledge the craving as a response to that emotion. "This craving is coming from a place of loneliness. I'll offer myself kindness and consider calling a friend instead of reaching for a drink."

3. Soften

Relax areas of the body that tense up during cravings. Physical tension often accompanies cravings, making it helpful to intentionally release this tightness.

» **Body scan:** Conduct a quick body scan to identify areas of tension. Common spots include the shoulders, jaw, belly, or hands. As you identify each area, consciously relax it.

» **Progressive muscle relaxation:** Tighten and then release muscle groups one at a time, starting from your feet and working your way up to your head. This practice can promote a deeper sense of relaxation.

» **Breath-focused softening:** Pair deep breathing with muscle relaxation. For instance, inhale deeply and, on the exhale, imagine warmth or softness flowing to the area of tension.

Example: If you notice tension in your shoulders during a craving, take a moment to lower them, breathe deeply, and let the tightness melt away. Repeat as needed until the physical urge diminishes.

4. Surround

Surround the craving with love and compassion. This final step involves treating the craving as something that needs care, rather than something to fight against.

> » **Visualization exercise:** Imagine the craving as a small child or a vulnerable part of yourself that needs comfort. Picture yourself holding it gently or surrounding it with a warm, compassionate light.
> » **Loving-kindness phrases:** Practice loving-kindness meditation by repeating phrases like, "May I be safe. May I be at peace. May I find comfort." Direct these phrases toward the part of you experiencing the craving.
> » **Welcoming the feeling:** Instead of trying to push the craving away, invite it in. Imagine opening your heart to the sensation and letting it exist without judgment. This acceptance can reduce the craving's intensity.

Example: When a craving arises, close your eyes and visualize it as a small child in need of comfort. Picture yourself embracing this "child" and offering it kind words, such as, "I'm here for you. It's okay to feel this way."

***

Dealing with cravings is one of the most difficult parts of becoming alcohol-free, but you can do it. It gets easier and easier as you progress on your journey. Keep working the 4S Model and you'll create a natural sense of joy in your life, even when things get tough.

THE RIPPLE EFFECT
OF THE ALCOHOL-FREE LIFESTYLE

With the toxins of alcohol gone from my body, I found that I started feeling good. Really good. And that inspired me to want to feel as good as I possibly could. Because I felt better, I started naturally becoming more interested in nutrition and exercise.

I started experimenting with the paleo lifestyle, working out regularly and ran a half marathon. I did a ten-day silent Vipassana meditation retreat outside Los Angeles and I even went to the infamous Burning Man festival, an annual week-long cultural event in Nevada's Black Rock Desert. (I was alcohol-free, of course). I did personal development workshops, including Landmark Education and a Tony Robbins seminar.

Making the commitment to my own health and happiness—which started with quitting booze—helped me become calmer and generate more peace and joy in my life. There tends to be a ripple effect here.

As soon as I eliminated my drinking habit, I found that it also unleashed a cascade of healthy habits that brought a deeper sense of contentment and joy flowing into my life. The biggest of those health habits was gratitude. I started living a life of appreciation rather than expectation. When I wasn't numbing myself with drinking, I became more present to the moments of my life—and a whole lot more grateful. It just happened naturally.

Another interesting observation I've made about the alcohol-free lifestyle is that it's something I can do for myself which genuinely benefits the people I care about most. It's a form of personal development that scales. When you make the commitment to stop drinking, it affects everybody you come into contact with—from the mailman, to the cashier at the grocery store, to your coworkers, friends, and family. You'll probably even treat your dog differently. You'll definitely treat yourself differently.

As a result of the clarity you begin to have without alcohol, you'll be able to listen and communicate better with everybody around you. You'll be more able to express your ideas, empathize with loved ones, and be more honest with yourself. This shift in the way you interact with others will improve their overall well-being, and they'll radiate that to others they come in contact with.

Some who notice your example will also follow in your footsteps because you may be the only person they've ever seen to voluntarily give up drinking. When people learn that you no longer need alcohol in your life, they are likely to question why they still feel the need to drink—and a certain percentage of those people may give it up for good. Your example might just be the final straw that broke the camel's back and nudged them in the direction of a complete life transformation.

Your decision to quit alcohol turns you into a radio tower that broadcasts positive, uplifting, and clear energy into a world that's often negative, depressing, and downright draining. That's something to be incredibly proud of.

You may never even know how you've helped people by simply existing, but it certainly is happening. People whom you inspire probably won't acknowledge you. In fact, they may not even remember it was your example that set them over the edge—and that's okay. Be confident that people are noticing. Some will judge you, but deep down, that's because the way you're carrying yourself reveals something threatening inside themselves.

Others will look at you and think of reasons why what you're doing wouldn't work for them. Show them through your clarity and consistency that the alcohol-free lifestyle is not magic. It's a scientifically proven system rooted in neuroscience. Then share this book with them and become accountability buddies.

IT'S TIME TO UNLOCK YOUR POTENTIAL

Choosing an alcohol-free lifestyle is more than just quitting drinking—it's an invitation to unlock a higher quality of life. When you eliminate alcohol, you clear the path to genuine fulfillment. The clarity and energy that come from a toxin-free mind and body inspire new pursuits and healthier habits, from improved nutrition and fitness to deeper mindfulness practices.

Without alcohol as a crutch, you'll learn to face life's challenges with courage, process emotions authentically, and cultivate resilience. This growth is contagious—your new habits, mindset, and energy influence everyone you encounter, creating a positive atmosphere that uplifts others.

Now is the time to reflect on your own relationship with alcohol. Ask yourself: What kind of life do I want to create? Am I ready to prioritize long-term fulfillment over short-term pleasure? If the answer is yes, then take that first step today.

Embrace the ripple effect that the alcohol-free lifestyle can bring, not just for your own sake, but for everyone around you. Your commitment to living with clarity, presence, and purpose will transform not only your life but also contribute to a world where genuine connection and sustainable joy become the norm.

Ready to begin your journey to becoming alcohol-free?
Get tools, support, and free resources at
www.alcoholfreelifestyle.com/resources

KEY TAKEAWAYS

» Alcohol numbs pain but blocks true healing—quitting allows you to face emotions
and grow.
» Pleasure is fleeting, but fulfillment lasts—
choosing growth over drinking leads to a
more meaningful life.
» Your choice to quit drinking inspires others
even if you don't know it, creating a ripple
effect of healthier, more conscious living.

CHAPTER 7 REFLECTION POINTS

Write out the answers to the following prompts in your
favorite journal to create simple, concrete action steps for
your alcohol-free journey.

Reflection: What activities, hobbies, or moments have
brought me genuine joy in the past, without alcohol?

Question: How can I redefine fun and fulfillment in my life
in ways that align with my alcohol-free goals?

Next Step: What is one joyful activity I can schedule this
week that doesn't involve alcohol?

"BEING ALCOHOL-FREE HELPED ME NAVIGATE MY GRIEF"

By Bill Cunningham
Federal Agent (Retired)
Eau Claire, Wisconsin

I WAS A LIFELONG DRINKER, AND for the past ten years, I was a heavy drinker. I was becoming extremely depressed, and my health was deteriorating. I didn't believe I could become alcohol-free and still be happy. I even developed alcoholic neuropathy in my feet. The doctor told me my feet weren't going to work anymore.

That was a wake-up call. I decided to stop drinking, and my health challenges cleared up quickly. Fast-forward one year, and I am a new person. I love being alcohol-free. My depression is almost nonexistent, and my health is back to normal. I feel great, both mentally and physically. Quitting alcohol was the best decision of my life. I will never drink that poison again.

In 2024, my father passed away. Being alcohol-free helped me navigate my grief. It has given me the gift of grieving my father with clarity. I love feeling the feelings, even though they can be painful. I have my life back.

CHAPTER 8:

YOUR STEP-BY-STEP ACTION PLAN TO BECOMING ALCOHOL-FREE

"Experience has taught me that there is one chief reason why some people succeed and others fail. The difference is not one of knowing but of doing. The successful man is not so superior in ability as in action. So far as success can be reduced to a formula, it consists of this: doing what you know you should do."

—ROGER BABSON

ACTOR WILL SMITH TOLD ME something when I interviewed him back in 2007 that I will never forget. He said, "When you set out to build a wall, don't think about the wall. Think about laying each brick as perfectly as a brick can be laid. And then you will have a wall." Similarly, starting the alcohol-free journey may feel overwhelming for some. But when you take it brick by brick, step by step, it becomes doable—and even easy.

At the end of this chapter, you'll find a 90-day "quick start" action plan to set a solid foundation for your alcohol-free lifestyle. Use this as your roadmap to stay on track in the beginning phase of your transition. Of course, I recommend that you turn your new habit into a lifelong pursuit of becoming clear and focused without alcohol—but you'll get there one day at a time. Ninety days is a good first milestone.

If you follow the steps, you'll be at Day 90 in the blink of an eye—and before you know it—Day 900. Let's lay those first bricks.

GET CLEAR ON YOUR "WHY"

You're nine chapters into this book, so it seems like a good place to pause and reflect. Why, exactly, do you want to be alcohol-free?

Getting extremely clear on this one question can lead to a series of breakthroughs in your ability to follow through on your commitment. Take the time to really consider why you want to live the alcohol-free lifestyle. Get a crystal-clear picture in your mind of how your life will tangibly improve when alcohol is no longer a part of it.

Here were a few of my "whys" for quitting alcohol:

» I wanted to lose that last stubborn ten pounds and get in better shape.
» I wanted to be more productive in my business and make more money.
» I wanted to improve the quality of my relationships and have deeper connections.
» I wanted to feel more in control of my life.
» I wanted to stop feeling so irritated over small problems.
» I wanted to wake up each morning with energy.

Once I embraced an alcohol-free lifestyle, each one of my reasons for starting the journey came true. The quality of my life tangibly improved every day I wasn't drinking. Since I had very strong "whys," it became easier to stay on track and generate amazing results. Thousands of our clients have found the same to be true on their alcohol-free journey.

As with any healthy changes in your life, results happen cumulatively.

Former research biochemist and author Robb Wolf framed it in a way that really resonated with me in his breakthrough book *The Paleo Solution*:

"Making the shift to a new lifestyle is challenging, but it's about taking it one step at a time and being consistent with your choices. You can't expect to change overnight, but with persistence, the results will come."[108]

Take the time to reflect on exactly what type of personal transformation you're looking to accomplish. Once you make the switch to living completely alcohol-free, you may experience a feeling of power and control over your life that you've never encountered before. This is how you'll know you're growing.

What would you like the freedom to do once you no longer feel the need to drink? I recommend you take the time to reflect on your deep and personal reasons for ending your relationship with alcohol.

You can make a list on your favorite notes application or in a word document. Sometimes, I even like to record a voice note to myself in order to talk through a scenario that's troubling me. Be as detailed as possible and brutally honest with yourself. Don't hold anything back—the purpose of the exercise is simply to create self-awareness.

Here are some examples of things you could write down:

- » *I want to get into the best shape of my life by age X.*
- » *I want to be a healthy and strong partner and parent.*
- » *I want to elevate my professional life and career.*
- » *I want to be highly paid for my work and recognized as top in my field.*
- » *I want deeper and more fulfilling friendships.*
- » *I want more love, intimacy, and connection in my relationship.*
- » *I want to be physically, mentally, and emotionally healthy.*
- » *I want to become more self-aware.*
- » *I want to feel more connected to a higher purpose.*
- » *I want to have power over my relationship with alcohol.*
- » *I want to break the generational curse of alcohol addiction in my family.*

As soon as you make the commitment to becoming alcohol-free, you're putting yourself in a better position to realize any future you can imagine by simply redirecting your energy into more beneficial habits and routines. By law of cause and effect, when you change where your attention goes, you'll change where energy flows, and where change ultimately takes place. Gradually, gradually, and then all at once, your new life will appear in front of you. When you see your ideal life starting to manifest, it will reinforce the fact that your decision to become alcohol-free was an excellent choice. That will be all the motivation you need to leave drinking behind.

REMOVING AND REPLACING ALCOHOL FOR GOOD

The physical space you live in has an outsized impact on your behavior. If you see alcohol, you're going to be triggered to drink. It's really that simple.

When I interviewed world-renowned habit change expert and author of the #1 *New York Times* best seller *Atomic Habits*, James Clear, during a private meeting with my students, he went into detail about exactly how you can change your environment to suit your goal of becoming alcohol-free.

Here's some of what he said in our fascinating conversation:

Your home environment can drive or dictate your habits in a variety of ways. If you walk into the kitchen and see a bottle of alcohol sitting on the counter, the visual stimuli that are triggers for your habit. How can we remove or reduce these triggers that are prompting alcohol consumption? One option is to throw the alcohol away. If you have alcohol, go ahead and just get rid of it immediately.

The second option is not to buy more of it. If you go to the grocery store, make sure you're not picking up additional alcohol. These options are extreme and they're going to work well, but they may not work in every situation. If you are in a situation where you need to keep alcohol in your environment, or your roommates bring it in or your spouse brings it back, then there are a couple things you can do.

In the fridge you can tuck the alcohol away in a less visible place. Whether that's far back on the top shelf, or far back on the bottom shelf, you want to have it in the back of the fridge so that you don't see it very well. You can also remove the number of visual cues that are at eye level, prompting the habit. If you have alcohol, go ahead and take it down from shelves that are near eye level and put it way down low or way up high. You can even put it in a box and store it in a different room. You can wrap it in tin foil, or put it in a bag.

Just make sure to remove the visual cue so that you don't
see it and you'll be much less likely to consume the alcohol.

Do you have a bottle opener in your kitchen drawer? Not anymore. Throw it away.

Do you keep a collection of corks from expensive wines you've tried? No, you don't. Toss 'em.

Remove the champagne glasses from view or give them away. Make your house feel as if alcohol never existed and you're one step closer to erasing it from your mind.

Next, find your replacements. Stock up on mineral water, sparkling drinks, tea, kombucha, or any other favorite alcohol-free drink and place it in your fridge. Then place a bowl of limes and lemons on the kitchen table so that when you see it each day, it reminds you to cut one open and squeeze it into your favorite alcohol-free drink.

I have my clients buy themselves a fresh bouquet of flowers, place it on their living room or kitchen table, and take care of it for a full week. The flowers become a symbol for your own body. The more you nurture the bouquet, the more you want to nurture yourself. Seeing the flowers daily will remind you of health, vitality, growth, energy, and color. This will help inspire you to make healthy choices, including remaining alcohol-free, exercising consistently, eating nutritious food, and doing things that help you grow.

You might also want to consider changing the media you're consuming if it doesn't support your commitment to remain alcohol-free. For instance, many commercials, television shows, and movies revolve around characters who are constantly drinking. Much of the music we listen to also promotes heavy drinking.

If you begin to take a mental tally of how often the media you consume references or directly encourages alcohol consumption, you'll be surprised at how often you're being bombarded with messages to drink alcohol. When you limit or eliminate the amount of programming you're taking in, it's much easier to stay focused on your goals.

In other words: guard your mind.

MAKING THE COMMITMENT

Once you've gotten crystal clear on your "whys" for leaving alcohol behind and you've cleared alcohol from your environment, you're officially in the game. Now it's time to commit to the lifestyle. That means you must make a conscious choice and follow through with action. Commitment is like a prism that focuses your energy onto whatever obstacle is in your way. When you align your thoughts and your actions, it gives you more power to accomplish whatever goals are in front of you. Everything will begin to flow more smoothly once you commit.

Motivational speaker and author Grant Cardone says, "Whenever you commit, you get immediate results. Whenever you're not committed, results are either delayed or nonexistent."

Changing your relationship with alcohol will require a commitment, there's no doubt about that. But the road to healing is counterintuitive. The truth is, healing doesn't always feel good, nor should it. The purpose of healing your relationship with alcohol is not because it will feel good or comfortable to do so—quite the opposite, in fact. Even with all the strategies I've outlined in this book, you'll still likely encounter many difficult emotions and conversations about your decision to become alcohol-free. I want you to run toward that feeling of discomfort and discover what you learn about yourself. Discover what you learn about society and the world as a result of your decision to become alcohol-free. Lean all the way in.

The nature of commitment means doing something for a greater purpose, because you promised yourself you would, regardless of how you feel in the moment. Commit to the lifestyle and reap the rewards. I recommend committing to the alcohol-free lifestyle for at least a year in order to really begin seeing the benefits. However, ninety days would be the minimum effective dose to experience the lifestyle.

In those ninety days, there is no retreat, no back-door way out. It doesn't matter if it's your birthday on day seventeen of your planned ninety days or if you're attending a wedding on day eighty-eight. You're all in.

A *Project 90* client once told me: "There was an evening during my challenge where I was tempted to drink. I was so close to my goal anyway, I thought, why would it matter? But I had that ninety-day number in my head and I knew I would be disappointed in myself for not reaching it."

How bad would you feel if you came so close to the end, only to throw it away at the last minute? Stay the course.

One thing that helped me in the beginning of my journey was to take it one day at a time. I didn't focus on the fact that I could "never drink again." Instead, I got excited about all the things I would be able to do now that I was alcohol-free. I had several opportunities to have a celebratory drink during the first year, and there were a few times when I strongly considered it. But after checking in with myself, I never felt like having a drink would actually make me feel any happier. So I just kept drinking club soda and lime... and before you know it, an entire year had passed. Then two, then five, then ten.

You don't necessarily have to swear off alcohol forever if you don't want to. You have free will. The goal may not be to declare you never can or should have a drink again. The goal is to make you aware of how easy it is to fall into the idea that you need to have a drink and to introduce the possibility that you can feel so good without alcohol that you never even question whether or not you should have it in your life. The problem solves itself as soon as you embrace the lifestyle and begin to see the results.

My advice after helping over 20,000 professionals get power over alcohol is: keep it simple. Don't overthink the process; trust the process. Remember what Will Smith says and lay the wall, brick by brick.

Before you know it, you'll have completed your mission.

GETTING COACHING AND ACCOUNTABILITY

In my experience of coaching people over the last decade, I've found that most people who try to use willpower to go alcohol-free on their own fail. You might have experienced trying and failing to quit one or more times yourself already. That's because it's extremely hard to do this alone.

One simple thing you can do right now to get accountability is to tell a family member, friend, or partner that you're committed to being alcohol-free and explain to them exactly why you're making this decision. Ask them if they'll support you and hold you accountable.

If you want to create bulletproof psychological leverage on yourself, try this:

Write a check to a charity or political candidate you despise for an uncomfortable amount of money. Seal it in an envelope, address it to the organization and put a stamp on it. Give the envelope to your accountability partner. Ask them to check in with you weekly for the next ninety days, and if you've had any alcohol at all, authorize them to drop the check in the mail. Then maintain your integrity by being honest with them when they ask.

Whatever method of accountability you choose, just know that it's nearly impossible to white-knuckle it and try to force your way through. There are powerful psychological factors at play with a habit that's become so deeply embedded. The most effective way I know to get ultimate power over your drinking is to do so with accountability from like-minded individuals. Ideally, you want to attempt your goal with people who are going through the same challenges as you and who will support and encourage you.

In the *New York Times* best seller *The Power of Habit*, Charles Duhigg says people only change when they are embedded in social groups that make change easier. "When people join groups where change seems possible, the potential for that change to occur becomes more real," Duhigg says. "For most people who overhaul their lives, there are no seminal moments of life-altering disasters. There are simply communities who make change believable."

This is the reason why our clients at Alcohol-Free Lifestyle succeed at such a high rate. In a recent study conducted by The University of Washington, participants in our *Project 90* stop-drinking program reported drinking 98 percent less over a period of ninety days—but this isn't because of any specific treatment we're providing. They are ultimately changing in response to a very specific community we have created.

Our programming is at the intersection of positive social engineering and self-improvement. The coaching from experienced professionals and the support from like-minded peers creates a perfect storm for positive habit change. You can't help but be transformed once you're in the vortex of positive energy and personal growth of AFL.

TIPS AND TOOLS FOR
CREATING ACCOUNTABILITY SYSTEMS

Below you'll find several examples for setting up accountability systems in one-to-one settings, small groups or privately with yourself. Choose the one that's right for you and stick to it.

1. Forming One-to-One Accountability Partnerships

Creating accountability partnerships is a powerful way to ensure you follow through with your commitment, but it can feel daunting (and even embarrassing) sometimes. Here's how to get started building your own accountability partnerships:

» **Choose the Right Partner:** Select someone you trust, who will be supportive but also firm in holding you accountable. This could be a friend, family member, coach, or mentor who understands your goals and is committed to helping you succeed.

» **Set Clear Expectations:** Discuss the specifics of your commitment. For example, agree on how often you'll check in (daily, weekly) and the type of support you need. Define what happens if you lapse in your commitment, such as your partner taking the steps outlined with the check to charity.

» **Use Scheduled Check-Ins:** Regularly scheduled check-ins are more effective than sporadic accountability. Use a calendar to set reminders for your check-ins, whether in person, via phone, or through video chat.

For example: "*Sarah and I agreed to meet every Monday morning for a coffee to discuss our weekly goals and check in on our progress toward staying alcohol-free. This keeps us both motivated and ensures we stay committed to our goals.*"

2. Joining Support Groups

Support groups can offer a sense of belonging and encouragement that is hard to find elsewhere. Here are some options:

» **In-Person Groups:** Many communities offer local support groups in person. These organizations provide regular meetings where you can share experiences and receive guidance.

» **Online Communities:** For those who prefer online interaction, there are numerous online forums, social media groups, and apps where people share their journeys and offer advice. Websites like Reddit's "r/stopdrinking" or Facebook groups dedicated to sober living are great starting points.

» **Structured Programs:** Programs like Alcohol-Free Lifestyle's *Project 90* offer a more structured environment, combining coaching, peer support, and resources tailored for people looking to cut down or eliminate alcohol.

Tip: When choosing a group, consider whether you prefer structured or flexible formats, anonymity or a more social atmosphere, and in-person or online connections.

3. Using Digital Tools and Apps

Leverage technology to enhance your accountability:

» **Habit-Tracking Apps:** Use apps like Habitica, Streaks, or HabitBull to monitor your alcohol-free progress. These tools allow you to set daily goals, track streaks, and receive reminders, keeping you focused on your journey.
» **Sober Living Apps:** Apps specifically designed for people cutting back on alcohol, like Sober Grid, I Am Sober, or Quit That provide daily motivation, community support, and personalized tracking.
» **Journaling Apps:** Use apps like Day One or Penzu to document your thoughts and feelings throughout your alcohol-free journey. Reflecting on your progress can help solidify your commitment and give you a sense of accomplishment.

YOUR "QUICK START" ACTION PLAN FOR BECOMING ALCOHOL-FREE

This "quick start" guide is designed to help you implement the principles outlined in this book over ninety days. Follow this simple, step-by-step timeline to begin your journey toward a healthier, more fulfilling life without alcohol.

Week 1 Checklist:
Preparation and Mindset Shift

1. **Set Your Intentions:** Start by understanding your reasons for going alcohol-free. Write down your "why." What do you hope to achieve by quitting alcohol (e.g., better health, more energy, improved relationships)?
2. **Clear Your Environment:** Remove all alcohol from your home and replace it with nonalcoholic alternatives. Stock up on healthy beverages like herbal teas, sparkling water, and alcohol-free mocktails.
3. **Create a Support System:** Inform your close friends and family about your decision and ask for their support. Join a community or support group where you can connect with like-minded individuals.
4. **Plan Your Triggers:** Identify your common triggers for drinking (stress, social events, etc.) and develop alternative activities or responses. For example, plan to exercise, meditate, or call a friend when feeling triggered.
5. **Mindset Exercises:** Practice daily affirmations and positive self-talk. Replace thoughts like "I need alcohol to relax" with "I enjoy my newfound clarity and peace."

Weeks 2 and 3:
Building New Habits

1. **Develop a New Routine:** Replace your usual drinking routine with healthier activities. If you used to drink after work, replace that habit with a walk, workout, or a relaxing bath, etc.
2. **Stay Busy and Engaged:** Fill your calendar with activities that keep you engaged and distracted from alcohol. Try new hobbies, take a class, or engage in creative projects.

3. **Monitor Your Progress:** Keep a journal of your feelings and experiences each day. Reflect on the positive changes you're noticing, such as better sleep, increased energy, and improved mood. Take progress pictures to track how your physical body changes.

4. **Stay Mindful in Social Situations:** Prepare for social events by bringing your own nonalcoholic drink or researching alcohol-free options. Practice confident and polite responses if offered a drink.

5. **Celebrate Small Wins:** Recognize and celebrate your progress, no matter how small. Each day alcohol-free is a victory. Reward yourself with something special—a favorite activity, a treat, or a new experience.

Weeks 4 through 6: Deepening Your Commitment

1. **Reflect and Reassess:** Take time to reflect on the changes you've experienced so far. Reassess your goals and reaffirm your commitment to an alcohol-free lifestyle.

2. **Strengthen Your Mindset:** Continue practicing positive affirmations and visualize your future without alcohol. Remind yourself of the benefits and how far you've come.

3. **Explore New Social Circles:** Start seeking out new social groups or activities that align with your alcohol-free lifestyle. Join a fitness class, attend a workshop, or participate in alcohol-free social events.

4. **Learn to Enjoy Socializing Alcohol-Free:** Experiment with enjoying social settings without alcohol. Focus on building deeper connections and being fully present in conversations.

5. **Stay Accountable:** Share your progress with your support network. Stay engaged in your community or support group to maintain accountability and motivation.

Weeks 7 through 9:
Overcoming Challenges

1. **Anticipate Challenges:** Identify potential challenges or temptations in the coming weeks and prepare strategies to handle them. Practice saying "no" with confidence and kindness.
2. **Deepen Your Self-Care:** Incorporate additional self-care practices to support your mental and emotional health. This could include regular exercise, meditation, yoga, or spending time in nature.
3. **Reconnect with Your Goals:** Revisit your "why" and reaffirm your reasons for quitting alcohol. Remind yourself of the benefits and positive changes you've already experienced.
4. **Focus on Personal Development:** Use this period to focus on personal growth. Read books, take online courses, or explore new hobbies that enhance your life without alcohol.
5. **Seek Professional Guidance if Needed:** If you encounter significant emotional or psychological challenges, consider seeking professional support from a therapist or counselor specializing in addiction.

Weeks 10 through 12:
Reinforcing New Habits and Celebrating Success

1. **Solidify Your New Lifestyle:** By now, your alcohol-free habits should feel more natural. Continue reinforcing these habits and building upon them.
2. **Reflect on Your Journey:** Look back on your ninety-day journey and reflect on your growth. Consider writing about your experiences, challenges, and triumphs in your journal.

3. **Plan for the Future:** Start thinking about your long-term goals for staying alcohol-free. What new habits or routines do you want to maintain? How will you continue to grow?

4. **Celebrate Your Achievement:** Celebrate your ninety-day milestone with a special activity or treat that rewards your commitment and hard work.

5. **Keep Moving Forward:** Understand that the journey doesn't end here. Continue building on the foundation you've created, and keep pushing yourself toward an even healthier, happier, and more fulfilling life.

✳✳✳

Remember, this journey is about progress, not perfection. Be kind to yourself, stay committed, and embrace the incredible benefits of an alcohol-free lifestyle. Your best life is just beginning.

> *Ready to begin your journey to becoming alcohol-free?*
> *Get tools, support, and free resources at*
> *www.alcoholfreelifestyle.com/resources*

KEY TAKEAWAYS

» A clear "why" keeps you committed—know your reason for quitting, whether it's better health, relationships, or productivity.

» Support and accountability make quitting easier—surround yourself with people who encourage your journey.

» Your environment shapes your habits—remove alcohol, add healthy alternatives, and minimize triggers.

CHAPTER 8 REFLECTION POINTS

Write out the answers to the following prompts in your favorite journal to create simple, concrete action steps for your alcohol-free journey.

Reflection: What has stopped me from succeeding in quitting alcohol in the past, and how can I approach it differently this time?

Question: What support systems or resources can I put in place to ensure my success in living alcohol-free?

Next Step: What is the first step I can take today to begin implementing my alcohol-free action plan?

"REMOVING THE SELF-LOATHING THAT HAD BECOME PART OF MY EVERY DAY"

Anna Lijphart
Nonprofit Founder and CEO
Alameda, California

EMBRACING AN ALCOHOL-FREE LIFESTYLE CHANGED my life. At the peak of my drinking, my weight was 184 pounds, but after I stopped drinking, I lost 30 pounds. I'm five feet ten inches tall, so the weight loss was huge for my self-esteem and self-confidence.

As an adult, I've always prided myself on my fitness—I'm a backpacking guide and avid hiker and mountain climber—but when my drinking spiraled out of control, so did my weight. Getting back to a healthy weight removed the self-loathing that had become a part of every day. Now, there is no longer a disconnect between my identity as a healthy and strong person and what I look like on the outside.

Project 90 freed me from the negative effects alcohol was having on my life. Every day, I'm grateful for the freedom, clarity, and intentionality I've gained by leaving alcohol in my rearview mirror. I look and feel better than ever.

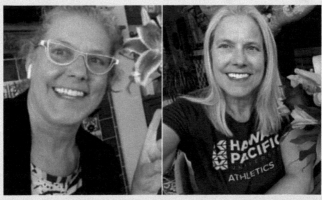

Anna lost 30 lbs and left self-loathing in the dust when she quit drinking.

CHAPTER 9:

EMBRACING THE UNCOMFORTABLE CLARITY OF YOUR NEW REALITY

"As an alcoholic, you will violate your standards quicker than you can lower them."

—ROBIN WILLIAMS

W HEN YOU STOP NUMBING YOURSELF with alcohol, you're going to feel more. Your mind is going to clear up very quickly. And although that's a good thing—the new reality you wake up to is not always going to feel like sunshine and rainbows.

Your newfound clarity might suddenly reveal years-long issues you've been deliberately suppressing, avoiding, or procrastinating on. People start seeing their lives—their relationships, career, and health—through a clear lens, when for years it was foggy.

World-renowned podcaster Jordan Harbinger shared his perspective on this transformation:

> I used to drink when I was younger as a social crutch. That habit continued into adulthood. Now, I don't need it and have cut alcohol out completely. It's one reason I'm in the best shape of my life at age 44. The sooner you stop drinking, the sooner you uncover what you need to work on. You can get to the root causes that are no longer masked. This is true personal growth and evolution.

One day, everything seems "normal." Then you stop drinking. You may start to realize:

"I'm in the wrong relationship."

"It's time to end my marriage."

"I shouldn't be in this job."

"I'm unhappy living here."

"I need to apologize to a certain person."

"I've been living a life of fear."

"I've wasted a decade."

These are scary realizations.

This chapter is all about dealing with the sometimes uncomfortable clarity of your alcohol-free life.

FINDING CLARITY IN YOUR RELATIONSHIPS

One client I work with, Lisa, ended a thirty-two-year marriage just six weeks into her first ninety alcohol-free days. She revealed to me she'd been pondering leaving the marriage for a decade. Going alcohol-free gave her the clarity and the courage necessary to accept that leaving the relationship was the right thing to do.

Did this feel liberating for her? Yes. But it also felt devastating.

"Sitting my husband down and telling him our marriage was over was one of the hardest things I've ever done," she said. "But it had to happen. Being alcohol-free finally helped me see that."

Only weeks after leaving the marriage, Lisa doubled down on herself by choosing to leave the family business to focus on her career. She was soon recruited by a Fortune 500 company for a role she absolutely loves.

"I really am grateful for the position I am in, as it has forced me to find a way to add more value to others," Lisa says. "Things couldn't have worked out much better for me."

Lisa's story is an example of how quitting alcohol "lifts the fog" from your life and makes it very clear in which direction you should head. So many people, me included, have spent years wasting time or energy heading in the wrong direction. When you quit alcohol, the answers to many of the most important questions about your life will become obvious—but that doesn't mean it'll be any easier to make the necessary changes.

At least now you'll always know which direction is your true north.

Recently, I was watching a video on author Mark Manson's YouTube channel in which he discussed his experience becoming alcohol-free after twenty-two years and how this change gave him clarity about which friendships were worth continuing. He said:

> In my thirties, I drank to bury my boredom. The epiphany I had when I stopped drinking is that if I'm bored when hanging out with certain people, I should simply stop being friends with those people. For some reason, this thought never occurred to me in the fifteen years that I was drinking, but now that I'm sober, it seems like the most obvious fucking thing in the world.[109]

Friendships can be very challenging to end—but romantic relationships can be even harder. If you've been in a romantic relationship for many years, it's likely that you are a different person now than you were at the beginning of the relationship. Choosing the alcohol-free lifestyle may affect your relationship.

Now that you're alcohol-free, it's a good time to reflect on your relationship. Here are a few questions to give you clarity:

» Do I feel seen, heard, and appreciated in my relationship?
» Am I able to communicate well with my partner?
» Do my partner and I help each other become healthier (mentally, physically and spiritually)?
» What's our sex and intimate life like?
» What are our family finances like?

Asking yourself questions like these and giving honest answers is the best way to get very clear about what you want out of your romantic relationship. If you find that your relationship isn't where you want it to be, you can choose to resolve it with your partner. You can have a clear, open and loving conversation about what you'd like to change and what your needs are. You can also hear their side and have empathy.

You can also choose to leave the relationship. You can have a clear, open and loving conversation about why you have to move on and what the next steps are. You can start the process of feeling happy again.

In your heart of hearts, you probably already know what the best choice for yourself is, so use the energy and clarity you've gotten back from being alcohol-free to do the work of repairing (or "retiring") your current relationship.

It goes without saying that as you reflect on your relationships, difficult truths may surface. Realizing you're in the wrong relationship or that a long-term partnership no longer aligns with your values can be painful. If these realizations lead you toward change, remember that it's okay to feel grief, relief, and everything in between. Take time to honor these feelings, knowing that they're valid.

Reflect on your relationship with compassion, and allow yourself to fully experience whatever emotions come up. Use this clarity as a tool for growth rather than a burden to carry alone. You're not only making decisions for yourself but also creating a life that reflects who you truly are—no longer blurred by alcohol's numbing effect. The path may be challenging, but you're stepping forward with integrity and courage.

STEPS FOR NAVIGATING DIFFICULT RELATIONSHIP DECISIONS

Reflecting on your relationships while alcohol-free can reveal whether a partnership is truly aligned with your values. Here's a structured approach to help you evaluate your relationship and start meaningful conversations.

1. Reflect on Your Feelings

Spend some time journaling about your relationship and answering the reflective questions in this chapter honestly. Write down both the positives and areas where you feel unfulfilled. This reflection helps organize your thoughts and emotions, making it easier to approach difficult conversations with clarity.

2. Prepare for the Conversation

When you're ready to discuss your thoughts with your partner, set the right tone:

- » **Choose a calm, private setting** where you both feel comfortable and free from distractions.
- » **Use "I" statements** to express your feelings without blaming your partner. For example, "I feel like I need more support in my health goals" is clearer and less accusatory than "You don't support me."
- » **Outline your objectives** before the conversation. Whether you want to work on improving communication, create mutual goals, or discuss the possibility of parting ways, being clear on your desired outcome can make the discussion more productive.

3. Listen Actively

Approach the conversation with empathy and openness. Ask questions to better understand your partner's perspective. For example, you might say, "How do you feel about where we're headed?" or "What are some ways we can support each other better?" Practicing active listening can lead to a deeper understanding of each other's needs.

4. Decide on a Path Forward

Based on the outcome of your discussion, decide together on the next steps:

» **If working on the relationship**, set mutual goals, such as regular check-ins, time set aside for shared activities, or counseling sessions.

» **If parting ways**, discuss a timeline and steps for handling shared responsibilities, financial matters, and the logistics of separation.

It's definitely not going to be easy, but taking these actions allows you to approach your relationship with honesty and courage, using your clarity to create a path that's truly aligned with your values and goals.

FINDING CLARITY IN YOUR CAREER

Deciding to go alcohol-free can bring up uncomfortable questions about whether or not you even like what you're doing for work. Worse yet, you might know that you actually hate your job—but you haven't done anything about it yet.

Clients I've worked with over the years have confessed to me that despite being well-respected and well-paid in their field, they were unhappy with their career for years. They've shared that giving up alcohol gave them the courage they needed to take the leap into new opportunities that were ultimately better for them—and just as lucrative, too.

Some self-help gurus will tell you that you should love your work so much that you'd do it for free if you could. Sounds nice in theory. In reality, I don't think anybody actually wants to work for free. We all want to be well-compensated for a job done well.

Here are a few questions to lend some clarity on the state of your career:

» *On a scale of 1 to 10, how much do I enjoy my day-to-day work?*

» *What would make it a 10?*

» *Do I feel like I'm using my unique interests and talents at work?*

» *Does it feel like there's an opportunity to grow in my career?*
» *Am I getting paid what I'm worth?*
» *Do I enjoy the people I work with?*
» *Am I proud of my work?*

We put so much energy into our careers, and to a large extent they reflect our chosen identity. It's worth stopping every few years to make sure you're on the right path and adjust accordingly. When something that you spend so much time on every day doesn't feel rewarding, exciting, or financially viable, you have to make a change.

Use your newfound clarity to dial in on your career path—and don't be afraid to make big changes. If you try something new and it doesn't work, it's likely that whatever job or field you left will still be there. But you'll never be able to go back in time and see how your career could have panned out if you'd just gone for what you really wanted.

If you've been investing time in a career that doesn't fulfill you, it's natural to feel frustrated. Allow yourself to experience these feelings without judgment. Recognize that every step in your career, even the ones that no longer serve you, has brought you to this point of insight.

As you consider change, trust that you're capable of navigating these decisions. Change is daunting, but your clear mind, strengthened by this journey, will guide you. You're not alone in feeling uncertain—many people have taken this leap and found greater fulfillment on the other side.

STEPS FOR NAVIGATING DIFFICULT CAREER DECISIONS

Going alcohol-free can often prompt reevaluation of your career path, especially if you find that your work is no longer fulfilling. Here's a practical approach to help you assess your career and consider new directions.

1. Assess Your Current Career Situation

Reflect on the questions in this chapter and rate your job satisfaction in each area. Consider factors such as day-to-day enjoyment, financial security, professional growth, and workplace relationships. Quantifying your level of satisfaction can clarify what needs improvement.

2. Explore New Opportunities Gradually

If you're considering a career shift but aren't sure where to start, try these incremental steps:

» **Network in fields of interest:** Attend relevant conferences, join online forums, or reach out to professionals on LinkedIn. This low-pressure way of learning about new industries can help you gauge if a career change is the right move.
» **Experiment with side projects:** Take on freelance work or volunteer roles that align with your interests. This allows you to explore new fields while maintaining the security of your current position.

3. Consider Necessary Training or Skills

If a new career requires specific skills or certifications, research potential courses or resources. Websites like Coursera, LinkedIn Learning, or Skillshare offer affordable online courses to help build relevant skills, providing a bridge between your current job and future opportunities.

4. Set a Timeline and Checkpoints

Establish a realistic timeline for when you'd like to transition fully. Set smaller milestones to keep yourself on track, such as completing a certification, applying for a certain number of jobs, or saving a financial buffer. Creating checkpoints helps you move forward with confidence and reduces uncertainty.

Changing careers takes courage, but it can lead to greater fulfillment. You'll never regret exploring your true potential.

CONFRONTING REGRETS AND TAKING RESPONSIBILITY

"Responsibility" is a curse word in the eyes of many people because it means being vulnerable enough to admit you were wrong—and it implies that you're ready to change. Alcohol can numb you to the poor decisions you've made or the careless ways you've treated others. When you stop drinking, those ghosts may come back to haunt you. It's easy to regret some of the things you've said or done when drinking was a regular part of your life.

If you really want to go back and open the past to apologize to people, I encourage that. This is a contentious issue and it's a personal choice you have to make in order to feel complete in your own healing process. Some people feel like they need to go back and acknowledge where they've done wrong. Other folks, like Christina Hansen, a New York City Central Park horse carriage driver and one of *Project 90*'s most successful clients, says, "Why would I ever do that?"

In a recent interview, Hansen added:

> "I think a lot of us (particularly women) drink because we don't want to hurt people, we want to be perfect because we're up against a lot of misogyny and told we need to behave a certain way. We don't want to go back and reopen old unhealthy wounds or behaviors. Maybe we drank for reasons like stress or escape that had nothing to do with having some sort of past trauma. We didn't crash a car, we didn't destroy our marriage or fuck up our children, we didn't hit rock bottom."

Fair point, Christina—and this is not Alcoholics Anonymous. You are not here to "make amends." However, if you choose to apologize to people for your past transgressions, the following section will give you a framework for doing so. The choice is yours.

Coming back to Mark Manson from earlier, he said it best in his book *The Subtle Art of Not Giving a F*ck*: "The more we choose to accept responsibility in our lives, the more power we will exercise over our lives. Accepting responsibility for our problems is thus the first step to solving them."[110] Being vulnerable in this way can be very hard at first, but it's the only way to be truly honest with somebody.

Taking accountability for past actions can be one of the most difficult aspects of this journey. You may feel guilt or regret for choices you made while drinking. These emotions are normal, and it's okay to feel them deeply. Instead of viewing your mistakes as a reflection of who you are, see them as opportunities for growth. Apologize to yourself for past choices and extend yourself the same compassion you would offer to a friend in your position.

When processing your regrets, remember that vulnerability is a sign of strength. If someone isn't ready to forgive, it doesn't diminish the power of your apology. True accountability lies in owning your actions and making a commitment to live with integrity moving forward.

STEPS FOR PROCESSING YOUR REGRETS

Healing isn't a linear process, but these are the basic steps for processing your regrets:

1. **Identify your regrets:** Make a list of past actions or words that you wish you'd handled differently. This could include relationships where there's lingering hurt or situations where you neglected responsibilities. Putting these regrets on paper helps clarify what steps you need to take to make things right.
2. **Reach out:** Reach out and apologize to those affected, if appropriate. Write a letter, schedule a conversation, or make a phone call to express your regret. Focus on taking responsibility for your actions rather

than expecting immediate forgiveness. If your actions caused harm, especially if financial or emotional, consider ways to make it right. This could mean reimbursing someone or providing additional support to repair the relationship.

If the person you'd like to speak with isn't available to receive your heartfelt apology (especially if they are no longer alive), there are other things you can do. Donate to a meaningful charity in their honor or dedicate something important to them.

3. **Forgive yourself:** Understand that everyone makes mistakes; the key is to learn from them and move forward. Then, define how you want to act going forward. Journal about the qualities you want to embody in your relationships and how you'd like to handle similar situations in the future. This commitment helps reinforce your decision to live with integrity.

4. **Create a plan:** Develop a plan to avoid similar mistakes in the future. Spend time regularly reflecting on your relationships by considering how you're showing up for others. Identify any areas where you could improve.

Just those four steps will give you much of what you need to know about popular stop-drinking programs and 12-step programs that have been around for decades. Facing areas where you hurt others and taking accountability is one of the most painful things you can do, but it's also one of the surest ways to know that you're growing. As you begin to turn a new leaf, you'll feel the weight of your past decisions begin to lessen.

Taking responsibility for past actions allows you to step into a new chapter with confidence, knowing that you're living in alignment with your values. This commitment not only repairs relationships but also strengthens your sense of self.

WINNERS GO AGAINST THE GRAIN

Going alcohol-free is going against the grain.

Never forget that there are powerful forces intent on stopping you from adopting the alcohol-free lifestyle. I'm not trying to sound like a conspiracy theorist—the truth is plain to see. Some of the biggest companies in the world spend billions of dollars every year to embed alcohol in every facet of popular media through advertisements, product placement, and more.

Remember, these companies wouldn't spend that much money unless it worked. They do it because they know that as long as their advertisements portray alcohol as being the gateway to fun, freedom, money, sex, or other positive emotions, people will continue to buy.

To defy this massive media assault on your mind is Herculean. Never forget what you're up against. You were already a top performer before you went alcohol-free. Now that you have taken this leap, you'll be unstoppable.

By now, you've hopefully realized that you don't need alcohol to enjoy social events. In fact, it can often be more fun to interact without it because you'll be clear enough to remember the details of all the celebrations and events you attend. Through the process of going alcohol-free you will break the mental link between alcohol and socialization. You'll no longer need it to connect with others.

As you continue on this path, your overall sense of joy and positivity will magnify. You'll have added many other things into your life which not only replace the high of alcohol, but also add to the overall quality of life. The temporary buzz of drinking is no match for the true satisfaction of feeling great and accomplishing your dreams over the long term.

Drinking often and heavily is the popular culture in most of the world—but the popular culture should not dictate your personal decisions. As it turns out, the more you lean away from popular culture, the happier your life becomes. The less you drink, the better you feel.

On a coaching call, one *Project 90* client said, "I've let alcohol control me. It's affecting my health, my family, and my ability to lead my business. It's killing my confidence and self-worth. I want to regain control and become the person I know I can be."

If that resonates, I can guarantee you this: Your self-esteem, confidence, and general outlook on life will transform when you go alcohol-free.

There will be times when making the decision to go alcohol-free is going to be challenging. You're going to have more than one good reason why it's okay to have "just one" drink. While I'm critical of the culture that champions alcohol, I'm not here to criticize individuals for drinking. We are products of our environments, and I was part of that culture at one time, too. Criticism is not how we've gotten thousands of clients inside the Alcohol-Free Lifestyle coaching programs to a greater than 90 percent success rate for nearly a decade.

There's nothing morally or ethically wrong with having a drink. There's also nothing wrong morally or ethically with ingesting rat poison, but you'd have to wonder why somebody would purposely poison themselves.

So, when it gets hard, don't forget your "why."

Your "why" could be to improve your mental and physical health. It could be that you want to improve your finances or marriage. Maybe your "why" is not having your kids grow up seeing you drink. Maybe it's because you're sick of getting passed over for a promotion every year. Find at least one emotionally compelling reason to embrace the alcohol-free lifestyle and lean into that when you're feeling weak and tempted to drink.

If you're ever tempted to have "just one," know that your struggle is part of the process. Be gentle with yourself and lean on your "why" to carry you through. The road to sustainable change isn't linear, but every challenge is a step toward becoming the person you're meant to be.

YOUR JOURNEY BEGINS NOW

For many people, efforts to stop drinking fall by the wayside simply because they focus on quitting for a short period of time, like thirty days. They tend to reach their goal and want to celebrate by—you guessed it—drinking.

It's easy to get discouraged if you keep trying to quit and failing—but there really is no such thing as failure when you're reprogramming your habits. All you need is time and consistency. If you fall, get back up again. The only thing that matters is that you're committed to starting over. Take it one day at a time.

You shouldn't think of being alcohol-free the same way you would think of a cultural phenomenon like Sober October or Dry January. This isn't about completing a "75 Hard" fitness challenge to prove to people on social media that you're cool. It's a powerful, personal life shift. It can also be a private one.

This is a years- or decades-long lifestyle, not simply a temporary event. My clients will often ask, "Can't I just drink on special occasions?" Well, the answer is yes. You are an adult, and you can do whatever you want.

But after all that you've learned...

Why are you still considering alcohol to be worthy of a special occasion?

As we've seen, alcohol is not special. Alcohol is not something to be desired. We've simply been socially conditioned to believe that it is. It's true that only drinking on special occasions is a massive breakthrough for those who are used to drinking every day after work. However, I invite you to rewrite the programming your brain has so readily absorbed and remove the notion that alcohol is special at all.

Let me ask you a single, profound question: "Is even one drink a day holding you back?"

After looking at the impact of alcohol from scientific, social and emotional perspectives, we've uncovered that the answer is undoubtedly a resounding "yes." But the power doesn't lie in the alcohol, it lies in you to make the necessary changes now that you have better information.

Now you know everything you need to know to take your power back from alcohol.

As you move forward, give yourself permission to feel the full range of emotions that accompany this new lifestyle. There is no single "right" way to go alcohol-free, so allow your journey to be unique. You'll have moments of doubt and times when you feel unstoppable. Both are part of the process, and every experience brings you closer to a life of clarity, fulfillment, and authentic joy.

Be proud of each step, no matter how small. You're not only breaking free from alcohol—you're creating a life that truly reflects who you are. This journey is challenging, but you're meeting it with strength, resilience, and compassion. Embrace the transformative power of this lifestyle, and trust that you're exactly where you need to be.

Now, take one concrete step. Choose one area of your life where clarity has revealed an opportunity for change, and create a plan. Outline small, achievable actions to begin addressing this area. Embrace this journey as a chance to live a life that is genuinely aligned with who you are becoming.

Ready to begin your journey to becoming alcohol-free?
Get tools, support, and free resources at
www.alcoholfreelifestyle.com/resources

KEY TAKEAWAYS

» Quitting alcohol brings clarity—though uncomfortable at times, it helps you see what needs to change in your life.
» Use this newfound awareness to face fears, make bold changes, and align your life with your true values.
» Change is an opportunity—set goals, take action, and design a life that truly fulfills you.

CHAPTER 9 REFLECTION POINTS

Write out the answers to the following prompts in your favorite journal to create simple, concrete action steps for your alcohol-free journey.

Reflection: What truths about myself or my relationships have I been avoiding by drinking, and how can I face them with courage?

Question: How can embracing discomfort lead to deeper growth and fulfillment in my life?

Next Step: What is one uncomfortable but necessary conversation or decision I can address to move forward?

"I FELT LIKE I WASN'T TAKING FULL ADVANTAGE OF MY ABILITIES"

By John Keltner
Sales Manager
Folsom, California

USED TO DRINK BEER AND whiskey, didn't sleep well, wasn't clear headed, and didn't look forward to getting up in the morning. I felt like I wasn't taking full advantage of my abilities and that alcohol was holding me back. I felt alone in this predicament.

I spoke to James about my problem, and he invited me to participate in *Project 90*, but I got nervous and declined, saying, "The holidays are starting; I'm going to wait until after the holidays."

He challenged me, asking, "Do you want to change your life?"

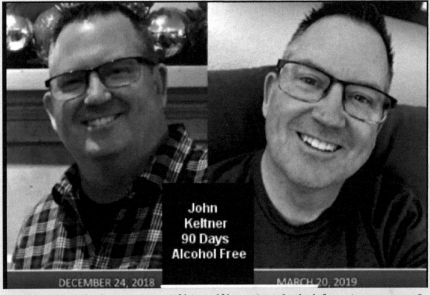

John
Keltner
90 Days
Alcohol Free

DECEMBER 24, 2018 ⸺ MARCH 20, 2019

John became the best version of himself by going alcohol-free. Are you next?

I said, "Yes."

Then he asked, "When would be a good time to start that?"

I replied, "I need to think about it. I don't make decisions like this without taking some time to really think about it."

James paused and then asked, "And how's that way of doing things working out for you?"

It was at that moment I thought, "Oh, he got me."

I realized I needed to take action, so I said, "Okay, James. I'm in."

Over the first ninety days, I went from 213 pounds to 195 pounds. I got down as low as 190 pounds a few months later. Over the last six years (2019–2025), I've maintained around 200 pounds. I feel healthy and athletic at fifty-nine years old, and of course, I'm still loving my alcohol-free life.

I even had to get slightly smaller glasses because of the loss of puffiness in my cheeks. Everybody compliments me on that, saying, "Oh, it looks like you've lost weight," and some even kid with me about looking skinny. Since quitting drinking, my life has changed for the better.

ACKNOWLEDGMENTS

THIS BOOK EXISTS THANKS TO the generous contributions of past and present Alcohol-Free Lifestyle (AFL) clients, teammates, mentors, friends, and family. It could not have been written without the support and dedication of many remarkable individuals, to whom I am eternally grateful.

First and foremost, I want to express my profound gratitude to my collaborator on this book, **Daniel DiPiazza**. Daniel, a friend since 2014, has brought tremendous value to the creation of CLEAR. His contributions were so significant that I insisted on acknowledging him on the book cover itself. Thank you, Daniel, for your outstanding work and for helping bring CLEAR to life.

Special thanks to:

» **My incredible AFL Executive Team (as of 2025)**: Adrian Nicholls and Becca Rolon, for your leadership and commitment to our mission.
» **Our extraordinary AFL coaches:** Victoria English, David Gilks, Teri Patterson, Matt Gardiner and Juliana Mendoza, for the unwavering support and guidance you provide to our clients.
» **The AFL Marketing Team, past and present:** Blake Chapman, Andrew Walton, Danny Seliger, Jeremy Haynes,

Chasen Gersh, Felix Millar, and Jeremy Van Dyke, for your creativity and efforts in sharing our vision with the world.

» **The AFL Enrollment Team:** Adam Hart, Sam Bizzell, Joel Brown, Jeff Dolan, Daniela Hogle, Chelsea Jamison, Neeshea Ho-Shing, and Brittany Vance, for your dedication in welcoming clients into our program.

» **My exceptional executive assistant:** Riza Samala, for your invaluable support since 2021 and for helping me stay focused and organized.

» **Former AFL teammates:** Kevin Schouweiler, Jim Miller, Felix Millar, Sarah Connelly, Michael Joseph, Zion Kim, Steve Costello, and Melanie Viaje, whose contributions have left a lasting impact on our mission.

I am deeply thankful to the business and personal development masterminds and programs I've participated in over the years. A special acknowledgment to **The Frontier Club**, of which I've been a member since 2011, for providing a lifetime of friends, advisors, and mentors, including Brent Sutherland, Leo Patching, and Peter Shallard. Additional thanks to **Jeremy Haynes** for his outstanding contribution to AFL's growth and impact; **James Schramko** for always going above and beyond with his support; and **Allyn Silver** with **Landmark Education** for inspiring me to be a better person and leader.

To **Tai Lopez**, my first entrepreneurial mentor: Thank you for your unwavering support over the years, for inspiring the creation of AFL in 2015, and for introducing me to an incredible network of friends, business partners, and collaborators.

To **Maya Burkenroad**, for your ongoing help over the years, and to **Mark Dhamma**, who inspired AFL's creation by encouraging me to sketch its first iteration on a Sunset Blvd hotel napkin in 2015.

Thank you to **David Belin**, Professor of Behavioral Neuroscience at Cambridge University, for his specialized research on impulsive and compulsive disorders, including alcohol and drug addiction. His work influenced some of our submissions in CLEAR.

To my dear friends: **Anthony McDonald, Mark Rutherford, Jason Rutherford, Thai Neave, Nico DiMattina, Kirk Westwood, David Kelly, Brad Blanks, Craig Hutchison, Andrew Collins, Juliana Mendoza, Claire MacNeill, Bob and Nadine Schramm, Bozho Deranja, Jerry Loeffler, Shane Martin, Chris Dufey, Maneesh Sethi**, and **Chris Melotte**—thank you for your friendship and encouragement over the years and decades. To my personal trainer, **Luis Tabla**, thank you for keeping me fit and healthy.

To the experts and friends referenced in CLEAR, including **Max Lugavere, Nir Eyal, Mark Manson, Keith Ferrazzi, Cory Muscara, Dan Go, Todd Herman, Jordan Harbinger, Dr. Michael Breus, Robb Wolf, John Gray**, and others—your work and insights have been invaluable.

To our incredible AFL clients, past and present, especially those who graciously proofread CLEAR during its creation and provided invaluable feedback, including **Christina Hansen, Danielle Hayden, Ronnie Bourgeois, Sheila Moore, Karen Grundhofer, Amy Venerable, Dawn Svedberg, Greg Stemler, Bill Cunningham,** coaches **Kannary Keo, Anna Lijphart, Steve Wilt, Evan Melcher, John Keltner, Robert Walsh** and **Jessica Gaines**—your support has meant the world to me.

To my parents, **Jill and Ron Swanwick**: Thank you for your unwavering love and support throughout my life. The values and morals you instilled in me have been the foundation for everything I do.

To my brothers, **Edward and Tristan Swanwick**: Thank you for being amazing Swanwick men and for bringing so much family comfort to my life over the years.

Finally, to my partner, **Laura**: You inspire me every day to be a better man. I love sharing this journey through life with you. Thank you for being my rock and my source of endless encouragement.

ABOUT THE
AUTHORS

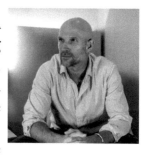

J AMES SWANWICK TRANSITIONED FROM A celebrated ESPN anchor to impacting thousands with his alcohol-free programs, showcasing a unique journey from media to coaching. As the founder of Alcohol-Free Lifestyle, and through his books and podcast, Swanwick has become a leading voice in health and wellness, inspiring millions to embrace a healthier, alcohol-free life.

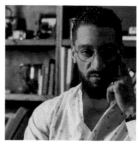

D ANIEL DIPIAZZA IS A BESTSELLING author and publisher at New Wave Press. His career has spanned multiple industries for almost two decades across film, television production, online education, coaching, new media, publishing and e-commerce.

He has dedicated his life to sharing his journey with millions of people around the world.

ALCOHOL-FREE

LIFESTYLE

GET SUPPORT FROM THE ALCOHOL-FREE LIFESTYLE COMMUNITY

Are you an executive or a top professional looking to stop drinking? Discover what it takes to REBOOT your life away from alcohol in 90 days.

If you're reading this book, there's a good chance that you'd be a fit for our *Project 90* experience, which helps high performers including business owners, leaders, entrepreneurs, real estate investors and top professionals like you stop drinking temporarily or permanently.

For some, that means never drinking again. For others, that means drinking modestly or on occasion.

In both scenarios, the *Project 90* experience has been helping hundreds of high performers get long-term control of alcohol.

With a proven plan, process and system that has a scientifically-proven 98% success rate, you'll be able to execute in 90 days what could take you years, maybe decades, of future struggle trying to get power over alcohol on your own.

To find out if *Project 90* is right for you, apply for a free consultation call with one of our experts at www.alcoholfreelifestyle.com/resources

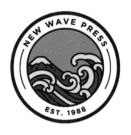

FOR ENTREPRENEURS, EXECUTIVES, AND PROFESSIONALS WHO ARE READY TO LEVEL UP THEIR CAREERS BY PUBLISHING A WORLD-CLASS BOOK

An expertly written, professionally published book is one of the best ways to position yourself ahead of the competition. It gives prospective customers a tangible reason to value your expertise, remember your name, and, ultimately, pay you more.

This book was published by New Wave Press, an "author-first" imprint that specifically caters to entrepreneurs and professionals who are ready to share their expertise with the world.

We take a true partnership approach. That means you get full creative control, access to the same caliber of production that traditional publishing offers — and you own your intellectual property forever.

Our job is to help you turn the credibility and authority from your book into a stepping stone that supports you in reaching your biggest goals.

It's all about you, as it should be.

To find out if you're a good fit to become the next New Wave author, schedule a call with our team at www.newwavepress.co/publish

TWENTY-TWO DELICIOUS ALCOHOL-FREE DRINK RECIPES

1. GINGER SPICE FIZZ

Ingredients:
- » Ginger ale
- » Agave syrup
- » Coriander
- » Cardamom
- » Cayenne
- » Orange peel
- » Rose oil

Instructions:
Mix ginger ale with agave syrup to taste. Add a pinch of coriander, cardamom, and cayenne. Garnish with orange peel and a drop of rose oil for a fragrant, spicy kick.

2. CRAN-LIME SPLASH

Ingredients:
- » Club soda
- » Splash of cranberry juice
- » Two lime slices

Instructions:
Pour club soda into a glass, add a splash of cranberry juice, and garnish with two slices of lime. Simple and refreshing!

3. CLASSIC SPARKLING LEMON WATER

Ingredients:
- » Sparkling water
- » Lemon
- » Ice

Instructions:
Fill a glass with sparkling water, squeeze fresh lemon juice into it, and add ice to chill.

4. TROPICAL MOCK-RITA

Ingredients:
- » Soda water
- » Splash of pineapple juice
- » Squeeze of lime

Instructions:
Pour soda water into a glass, add a splash of pineapple juice and a squeeze of lime. Stir and enjoy this margarita-like mocktail.

5. PERRIER CRANBERRY

Ingredients:
- » Perrier
- » Cranberry juice

Instructions:
Simply pour Perrier into a glass and add cranberry juice. Enjoy it straight for a clean and simple mocktail.

6. VIRGIN MOJITO

Ingredients:
- » Mint leaves
- » Ice
- » Seltzer
- » Lime

Instructions:
Muddle mint leaves with ice in a glass. Add seltzer and a squeeze of lime for a refreshing virgin mojito.

7. CLEANSING GINGER-CUCUMBER-MINT DRINK

Ingredients:
- » Ginger
- » Cucumbers
- » Mint leaves
- » Water

Instructions:
Add slices of ginger, cucumber, and fresh mint leaves to a pitcher of water. Let it steep overnight for a refreshing and cleansing drink.

8. SPARKLING CRANBERRY-LIME WATER

Ingredients:
- » Sparkling water
- » Cranberry juice
- » Lime

Instructions:
Fill a glass with sparkling water, add cranberry juice, and top with a slice of lime for a refreshing mocktail.

9. MINTY SELTZER

Ingredients:
- » Mint leaves
- » Ice
- » Seltzer
- » Lime

Instructions:
Muddle mint leaves and ice, pour seltzer over, and garnish with a squeeze of lime for a crisp and minty drink.

10. CRANBERRY FIZZ

Ingredients:
- » Cranberry juice
- » Sparkling water
- » Ice

Instructions:
Mix cranberry juice with sparkling water, add ice, and enjoy this simple, refreshing drink.

11. HOT HONEY TEA

Ingredients:
- » Tea of your choice
- » Honey

Instructions:
Brew your favorite tea, stir in honey, and enjoy a soothing, dopamine-boosting beverage.

12. NON-ALCOHOLIC BEER & SPARKLING WATER

Ingredients:
- » Non-alcoholic beer
- » Sparkling water
- » Grapefruit slices (optional)

Instructions:
Pour non-alcoholic beer and sparkling water into a glass, and garnish with grapefruit slices for an interesting and refreshing twist.

13. SPECIALTY INFUSED SPARKLING WATER

Ingredients:
- » Sparkling water
- » Lavender or cucumber infusion

Instructions:
Add your choice of lavender or cucumber infusion to sparkling water for a light, aromatic drink.

14. SPARKLING ROSÉ MOCKTAIL

Ingredients:
 » Sparkling rosé 0%
 » Apple cider

Instructions:
Pour sparkling rosé 0% into a glass, then top with apple cider for a celebratory mocktail served in a champagne glass.

15. CLASSIC CIDER

Ingredients:
 » Cider (alcohol-free)

Instructions:
*Pour your favorite non-*alcoholic cider into a glass and enjoy this refreshing, sweet drink.

16. FLAVORED SODA WATER OR KOMBUCHA

Ingredients:
 » Flavored soda water (e.g., Canada Dry) or your favorite kombucha

Instructions:
Chill and pour into a glass. No extra ingredients needed for these refreshing drinks.

17. APPLE-CUCUMBER-CELERY SMOOTHIE

Ingredients:
 » Apple
 » Cucumber
 » Celery
 » Protein powder
 » Coconut water

Instructions:
Blend apple, cucumber, and celery with protein powder and coconut water. Add ice for a smooth, filling drink that can also serve as a meal.

18. CRANBERRY SUNRISE SPARKLER

Ingredients:
- » Cranberry juice (100%)
- » Orange juice
- » Sparkling water

Instructions:
Mix 100% cranberry juice with orange juice and sparkling water for a tart and fizzy drink.

19. GINGER ALE AND LEMON

Ingredients:
- » Ginger Ale
- » Lemon

Instructions:
Pour ginger ale into a glass and squeeze lemon. Enjoy a flavorful, non-alcoholic soda.

20. CHERRY POMEGRANATE SELTZER

Ingredients:
- » Pomegranate seltzer water
- » Tart cherry juice
- » Lime
- » Ice

Instructions:
Pour pomegranate seltzer and tart cherry juice into a glass. Add a squeeze of lime and lots of ice for a refreshing, calming drink.

21. LIME-CUCUMBER-MINT WATER

Ingredients:
- » Soda water
- » Lime
- » Cucumber slices
- » Mint

Instructions:
Pour soda water into a glass, add a slice of lime, cucumber slices, and mint for a fresh and rejuvenating drink.

22. CRANBERRY BERRY SMASH

Ingredients:
- » Soda water
- » Cranberry juice
- » Frozen berries (rasp-
  berries, blueberries,
  blackberries)

Instructions:
Mix soda water with cranberry juice, and add frozen berries. Smash them lightly to release the flavor, and enjoy.

APPENDIX B

AFL RESEARCH STUDY

EFFECT OF *PROJECT 90* PARTICIPATION ON SELF-REPORTED ALCOHOL CONSUMPTION

Christopher M. Barnes
University of Washington

Shawn Quan
University of Washington

Mo Wang
University of Florida

J. Jeffrey Gish
University of Central Florida

EXECUTIVE SUMMARY

Project 90 is a 90-day intervention program developed by Alcohol-Free Lifestyle, aimed at fostering sustainable changes in alcohol consumption behaviors through a blend of coaching, social support, and behavioral exercises. This study explored the effectiveness of *Project 90* through a carefully designed field experiment involving 164 participants who reported a pre-study alcohol consumption rate of 19 drinks per week. Participants were randomly assigned to either begin *Project 90* at the beginning of the study or after the final survey of the study (waitlist control group). The final survey of the study was 60 days into the study. Participants in the *Project 90* program participation group reported an average of just 0.03 alcoholic drinks per day, in contrast to the waitlist control group's average of 1.52 drinks per day. In other words, self-reported drinking was 98% less for those who were participating in the *Project 90* program than in those in the waitlist control group. Furthermore, the *Project 90* program participation group reported drinking on only 3% of the study days, compared to 48% in the waitlist control group.

INTRODUCTION

Alcohol-Free Lifestyle is an organization which has a treatment program intended to help high performers take back control of their drinking. Among their programs is *Project 90*, which is a 90-day program composed primarily of coaching, social support, and behavioral exercises. The intention behind the program is sustainable change in alcohol consumption. For further details about Alcohol-Free Lifestyle and *Project 90*, please consult their materials.

The author team (Quan, Barnes, Wang, and Gish) partnered with Alcohol-Free Lifestyle to conduct a study of the efficacy of *Project 90*. It is worth noting that this author team has no financial entanglements with Alcohol-Free Lifestyle, nor any other non-financial arrangements beyond simply conducting this study. For the author team, the intention was to conduct a scientific investigation of the effects of an alcohol consumption change program with the type of format that *Project 90* has. For Alcohol-Free Lifestyle, the intention was to have independent third party researchers test the efficacy of *Project 90*.

This report documents the result of the study. In the following sections, we discuss the research method (including the research design and the measures), the results, and close with a brief discussion.

METHOD
Participants

A total of 164 participants were recruited to participate in the study. Participants were recruited by *Project 90* staff at the beginning of their consultation. Out of all participants, 109 (2/3 of total) were randomly assigned to the treatment condition, while 55 (1/3 of total) were assigned to be in the waitlisted control condition. After data validation checks, a total of 157 participants passed the validation and are presented in the final sample.

Participants are from a diverse range of geographic locations, with the largest portions of participants from the United States, Australia, and Germany. 89% of the participants were white, and 51% were male. The average age of participants was 49 years old. On average, participants worked remote half of their total workdays. Before the study started, participants consumed an average of 19 alcoholic drinks per week.

RESEARCH DESIGN

In this study, we conducted a field experiment with random assignment of participants to either participate in *Project 90* at the beginning of the study (we refer to this group as the "Treatment" group) or remain in a waitlist for 60 days and then begin *Project 90* (we refer to this group as the "Control" group). In both conditions, participants began the study at the same time. In other words, Treatment and Control participants completed surveys at the same time, but Treatment participants were working through *Project 90* during the course of those surveys, and Control participants did not begin *Project 90* until after completing the final survey of our study. This allowed us to compare the effects of those actively engaged in *Project 90* with those who were not, with random assignment of participants to conditions minimizing the initial differences between those two groups.

Creating this research design required a balance between trying to measure relatively long-term outcomes from *Project 90* against the concern about making people in the waitlist group wait too long to participate in the program. Ultimately, we decided that the best balance among these goals was to aim for a 60-day period for the waitlist. This meant that although *Project 90* is a 90-day program, our study stopped observing participants after 60 days.

The study was conducted from January to March 2023. Participants started with an entry survey that measured their demographic information and baseline drinking habits. Starting on day 45 of the study, participants receive two daily diary surveys a day, for 14 consecutive days. These surveys asked for participants' daily workload, mood, drinking behavior, and daily behaviors at work, such as helping their coworkers and their work engagement. Participants receive the morning survey at the beginning of their work day (6 am) and the evening survey at the end of their work day (6 pm).

Overall, a total of 29 surveys were sent out per employee. The average response rate is 61% (99% for the entry survey, 77% for the longitudinal surveys, and 53% for the daily diary surveys).

The outcome of interest in this study was alcohol consumption. To measure alcohol consumption, we first established the baseline of their alcohol consumption behavior in the entry survey by asking the frequency and average number of alcoholic drinks they consume in a typical week before the start of the study. During the study, we asked participants the following question in their evening surveys at the end of day: "How many alcoholic drinks did you consume today?"

RESULTS

Overall, we found a statistically significant difference between the treatment and waitlisted group in alcohol consumption. After six weeks of treatment, participants who were in the treatment group reported consuming an average of 0.03 alcoholic drinks/day, while those in the waitlisted group reported consuming an average of 1.52 alcoholic drinks/day. In other words, self-reported drinking was 98% less for those who were participating in the Project 90 program than in those in the waitlist control group. Those in the treatment group reported drinking on only 3% of study days, while those in the waitlisted group reported drinking on 48% of study days. Given the clustered nature of the data (days nested within person), we conducted a multilevel regression analysis. This analysis indicated that being in the treatment group significantly decreased participants' self-reported daily alcohol consumption ($B = -1.48$, $SE = 0.19$, $p < 0.01$).

Group	Total person*days without drinking	Total person*days	Percentage of Days Without Alcohol
Waitlisted	223	468	0.48
Treatment	691	712	0.97

Figure 1: Comparison of Alcohol Consumption

DISCUSSION

In this study, the evidence was clear that participants reported less drinking in the Treatment group than the Control group. In other words, those assigned to receive *Project* 90 immediately reported consuming less alcohol than those who had not yet begun *Project* 90. This evidence suggests that *Project* 90 helps people to lower their alcohol consumption.

There are three important limitations of this study worth noting. One is that our research design cannot rule out the possibility of a placebo effect. Because of the practical limitations of conducting this sort of a study, neither participants in the Treatment condition nor those in the Control condition were blind to which condition they were assigned to. Knowing which condition they were assigned to opens up the possibility that their beliefs about the treatment (or lack thereof) could influence their responses above and beyond any objective effects. A second limitation is that our measure of alcohol consumption was a self-report measure. This was again a practical limitation of conducting this sort of field experiment. We had no objective measures of alcohol consumption, and we cannot rule out the possibility that participants lied about their alcohol consumption. Specifically, we cannot rule out the possibility that participants under-reported their alcohol consumption.

The final limitation is simply that our study entailed a specific time window. We believe that our time window ends at 60 days into the study time frame for this study. However, we have no data about participants beyond the final survey of the study. We cannot make any statements about the efficacy of *Project* 90 beyond the period of observation in our study.

We hope that future research follows up on this study and addresses the specific limitations of our study, and eliminates any remaining uncertainties. Nevertheless, our independent assessment is cautiously optimistic that *Project* 90 is effective in helping participants to lower their alcohol consumption.

NOTES

Introduction

[1] National Institute on Alcohol Abuse and Alcoholism. «Understanding Alcohol Use Disorder.» National Institute on Alcohol Abuse and Alcoholism, U.S. Department of Health and Human Services, www.niaaa.nih.gov/publications/brochures-and-fact-sheets/understanding-alcohol-use-disorder.

[2] Boersma, Peter, Maria A. Villarroel, and Anjel Vahratian. «Products - Data Briefs - Number 374- August 2020.» Centers for Disease Control and Prevention, August 2020, www.cdc.gov/nchs/products/databriefs/db374.htm.

[3] American Psychiatric Association. *Diagnostic and Statistical Manual of Mental Disorders.* 5th ed., American Psychiatric Publishing, 2013.

Why We Drink

[4] Daviet, Remi, et al. «Associations Between Alcohol Consumption and Gray and White Matter Volumes in the UK Biobank.» *Nature Communications* 13, no. 1 (2022): 1175.

[5] Eyal, Nir. *Hooked: How to Build Habit-Forming Products.* Penguin, 2019.

[6] Duhigg, Charles. *The Power of Habit: Why We Do What We Do, and How to Change.* Random House, 2013.

[7] Rehm, Jürgen, and Kevin D Shield. "Global Burden of Alcohol Use Disorders and Alcohol Liver Disease." *Biomedicines* vol. 7,4 99. 13 Dec. 2019, doi:10.3390/biomedicines7040099.

[8] Walsh K, Alexander G. Alcoholic liver disease. *Postgrad Med J.* 2000 May;76(895):280–6. doi: 10.1136/pmj.76.895.280. PMID: 10775280; PMCID: PMC1741594.

[9] Smith, Sarah. "What Alcohol Does to Your Body After 40." *Sydney Morning Herald,* 15 Dec. 2015, www.smh.com.au/lifestyle/health-and-wellness/what-alcohol-does-to-your-body-after-40-20151215-glnhek.html. Accessed 20 Aug. 2024.

[10] Briasoulis, Alexandros et al. "Alcohol consumption and the risk of hypertension in men and women: a systematic review and meta-analysis." *Journal of Clinical Hypertension (Greenwich, Conn.)* vol. 14,11 (2012): 792–8. doi:10.1111/jch.12008.

[11] Cecchini, Marta et al. "Alcohol Intake and Risk of Hypertension: A Systematic Review and Dose-Response Meta-Analysis of Nonexperimental Cohort Studies." *Hypertension* (Dallas, Tex., 1979) vol. 81,8 (2024): 1701–1715. doi:10.1161/HYPERTENSIONAHA.124.22703.

[12] Larsson, Susanna C et al. "Differing association of alcohol consumption with different stroke types: a systematic review and meta-analysis." *BMC medicine* vol. 14,1 178. 24 Nov. 2016, doi:10.1186/s12916-016-0721-4.

[13] International Diabetes Federation. *Diabetes Atlas,* 10th ed., International Diabetes Federation, 2021.

[14] Bagnardi V, Rota M, Botteri E, et al. "Alcohol consumption and site-specific cancer risk: A comprehensive dose-response meta-analysis." *British Journal of Cancer* 2015; 112(3):580–593.

[15] Chen WY, Rosner B, Hankinson SE, Colditz GA, Willett WC. "Moderate alcohol consumption during adult life, drinking patterns, and breast cancer risk." JAMA 2011; 306(17):1884–1890.

[16] International Agency for Research on Cancer. IARC Monographs on the Identification of Carcinogenic Hazards to Humans: Agents Classified by the IARC Monographs, Volumes 1–136. World Health Organization, 2024, https://monographs.iarc.who.int/agents-classified-by-the-iarc/. Accessed 20 Aug. 2024.

[17] Sullivan, Edith V., et al. "Alcohol Drinking and Alcohol Use Disorder Across the Ages: Dynamic Effects on the Brain and Function." APA Handbook of Neuropsychology, vol. 1, American Psychological Association, 2023. Springer.

[18] Swendsen, J., Merikangas, K., Canino, G., et al (1998). The comorbidity of alcoholism with anxiety and depressive disorders in four geographic communities. Comprehensive Psychiatry, 39, 176–184.

[19] Pohl, Keith et al. "Alcohol›s Impact on the Gut and Liver." Nutrients vol. 13,9 3170. 11 Sep. 2021, doi:10.3390/nu13093170.

[20] "Overview of Malabsorption." The Merck Manual of Diagnosis and Therapy, Merck & Co., Inc., 2023, https://www.merckmanuals.com/professional/gastrointestinal-disorders/malabsorption-syndromes/overview-of-malabsorption.

[21] Goodman, Greg D et al. "Impact of Smoking and Alcohol Use on Facial Aging in Women: Results of a Large Multinational, Multiracial, Cross-sectional Survey." The Journal of Clinical and Aesthetic Dermatology vol. 12,8 (2019): 28–39.

[22] Liu, Lin, and Jin Chen. "Advances in Relationship Between Alcohol Consumption and Skin Diseases." Clinical, cosmetic and investigational dermatology vol. 16 3785-3791. 29 Dec. 2023, doi:10.2147/CCID.S443128.

[23] Li, Shen et al. "A Meta-Analysis of Erectile Dysfunction and Alcohol Consumption." Urologia internationalis vol. 105,11-12 (2021): 969-985. doi:10.1159/000508171.

[24] Peugh, J, and S Belenko. "Alcohol, drugs and sexual function: a review." Journal of Psychoactive Drugs vol. 33,3 (2001): 223–32. doi:10.1080/02791072.2001.10400569.

[25] Emanuele, Mary Ann et al. "Alcohol›s effects on female reproductive function." Alcohol Research & Health: The Journal of the National Institute on Alcohol Abuse and Alcoholism vol. 26,4 (2002): 274–81.

[26] Shield, Kevin D et al. "Alcohol Use and Breast Cancer: A Critical Review." Alcoholism, Clinical and Experimental Research vol. 40,6 (2016): 1166–81. doi:10.1111/acer.13071.

[27] Centers for Disease Control and Prevention. "Deaths from Excessive Alcohol Use—United States, 2016–2021." MMWR, 2021, www.cdc.gov. Accessed 8 Oct. 2024.

[28] Taylor, Mark et al. "Quantifying the RR of harm to self and others from substance misuse: results from a survey of clinical experts across Scotland." BMJ Open vol. 2,4 e000774. 24 Jul. 2012, doi:10.1136/bmjopen-2011-000774.

[29] "Ranking the Harm of Psychoactive Drugs Including Prescription Analgesics to Users and Others—A Perspective of German Addiction Medicine Experts." Frontiers in Psychiatry, vol. 8, 2017, doi:10.3389/fpsyt.2017.00129.

[30] David Nutt, A Risky Business? Comparing the Harms of Alcohol and Other Recreational Drugs, Significance, vol. 18, Issue 2, April 2021, pages 40–42, https://doi.org/10.1111/1740-9713.01512

[31] Ritchie, Hannah, and Max Roser. «Share of Road Traffic Deaths Attributed to Alcohol.» Our World in Data, Global Change Data Lab, 3 Jan. 2024, ourworldindata.org/grapher/road-traffic-deaths-to-alcohol. Accessed 9 Oct. 2024.

[32] Greenfield, Ben. "What Alcohol Really Does to Your Body, Brain, and Spirit." Ben Greenfield Life, 22 July 2021, bengreenfieldlife.com/podcast/alcohol-podcast/. Accessed 20 Aug. 2024.

[33] Dodes, Lance, and Zachary Dodes.*The Sober Truth: Debunking the Bad Science behind 12-Step Programs and the Rehab Industry. Beacon Press, 2014.

[34] American Addiction Centers. "Drug Rehab Success Rates and Statistics." American Addiction Centers, 20 Aug. 2023, americanaddictioncenters.org/rehab-guide/success-rates-and-statistics. Accessed 20 Aug. 2024.

[35] Barnes, Christopher M., et al. *Effect of Project 90 Participation on Self-Reported Alcohol Consumption.* University of Washington, University of Florida, University of Central Florida, 2023.

How to Refocus Your Mindset Around Alcohol

[36] Holiday, Ryan. *The Obstacle Is the Way: The Timeless Art of Turning Trials into Triumph.* Portfolio/Penguin, 2014.

[37] Helmstetter, Shad. *What to Say When You Talk to Yourself.* Park Avenue Press, 1982

[38] Brocardo, Patricia S., et al. "Exploring the Role of Neuroplasticity in Development, Aging, and Neurodegeneration." *Brain Sciences*, vol. 13, no. 12, 2023, p. 1610, https://doi.org/10.3390/brainsci13121610. Accessed 21 Nov. 2023.

[39] Shaffer, J. (2012). "Neuroplasticity and Positive Psychology in Clinical Practice: A Review for Combined Benefits." *Psychology*, 3, 1110-1115. doi: 10.4236/psych.2012.312A164.

[40] Casico, Christopher N., Matthew Brook O'Donnell, Francis J. Tinney, Matthew D. Lieberman, Shelley E. Taylor, Victor J. Strecher, Emily B. Falk, "Self-affirmation activates brain systems associated with self-related processing and reward and is reinforced by future orientation," *Social Cognitive and Affective Neuroscience*, vol. 11,4, April 2016, pages 621–629, https://doi.org/10.1093/scan/nsv136

[41] Hebb, D.O. *The Organization of Behavior: A Neuropsychological Theory.* 1st ed., Wiley, 1949.

[42] Taran, Shaurya et al. "The reticular activating system: a narrative review of discovery, evolving understanding, and relevance to current formulations of brain death." *Canadian Journal of Anesthesia* vol. 70,4 (2023): 788-795. doi:10.1007/s12630-023-02421-6

[43] Clear, James. *Atomic Habits: An Easy & Proven Way to Build Good Habits & Break Bad Ones.* Avery, 2018.

[44] Giannone, Fabio, et al. "Bad Habits-Good Goals? Meta-analysis and Translation of the Habit Construct to Alcoholism," *Translational Psychiatry.*

[45] Corbin, William R et al. "Contextual influences on subjective alcohol response." *Experimental and Clinical Psychopharmacology* vol. 29,1 (2021): 48–58. doi:10.1037/pha0000415.

[46] Koob, George F, and Nora D Volkow. "Neurobiology of addiction: a neurocircuitry analysis." *The Lancet. Psychiatry* vol. 3,8 (2016): 760–773. doi:10.1016/S2215-0366(16)00104-8.

[47] Mehrabian, Albert. *Silent Messages: Implicit Communication of Emotions and Attitudes.* Wadsworth Publishing Company, 1971.

[48] Ferrazzi, Keith, and Tahl Raz. *Never Eat Alone: And Other Secrets to Success, One Relationship at a Time.* Expanded and Updated ed., Crown Business, 2014. Amazon.

[49] Herman, Todd. *The Alter Ego Effect: Defeat the Enemy, Unlock Your Heroic Self, and Start Kicking Ass.* Harper Business, 2019.

Healing the Effects of Alcohol on Your Brain and Body

[50] "The Surprising Ways Alcohol is Ruining Your Life," *The Genius Life*, hosted by Max Lugavere, episode 51, 23 Aug. 2024.

[51] León, Brandon Emanuel et al. "Alcohol-Induced Neuroinflammatory Response and Mitochondrial Dysfunction on Aging and Alzheimer›s Disease." *Frontiers in Behavioral Neuroscience* vol. 15 778456. 10 Feb. 2022, doi:10.3389/fnbeh.2021.778456.

[52] Zahr, Natalie M, and Adolf Pfefferbaum. "Alcohol›s Effects on the Brain: Neuroimaging Results in Humans and Animal Models." *Alcohol Research: Current Reviews* vol. 38,2 (2017): 183–206.

[53] Zahr, Natalie M, and Adolf Pfefferbaum. "Alcohol›s Effects on the Brain: Neuroimaging Results in Humans and Animal Models." *Alcohol Research: Current Reviews* vol. 38,2 (2017): 183–206.

[54] Volkow, Nora D et al. "Profound decreases in dopamine release in striatum in detoxified alcoholics: possible orbitofrontal involvement." *The Journal of Neuroscience: The Official Journal of the Society for Neuroscience* vol. 27,46 (2007): 12700-6. doi:10.1523/JNEUROSCI.3371-07.2007.

[55] Davies, Martin. "The role of GABAA receptors in mediating the effects of alcohol in the central nervous system." *Journal of Psychiatry & Neuroscience: JPN* vol. 28,4 (2003): 263–74.

[56] Banerjee, Niladri. "Neurotransmitters in alcoholism: A review of neurobiological and genetic studies." *Indian Journal of Human Genetics* vol. 20,1 (2014): 20–31. doi:10.4103/0971-6866.132750.

[57] Emmons, Robert A., and Michael E. McCullough. "Counting blessings versus burdens: an experimental investigation of gratitude and subjective well-being in daily life." *Journal of Personality and Social Psychology* vol. 84,2 (2003): 377–89. doi:10.1037//0022-3514.84.2.377.

[58] McCraty, R. et al. "The impact of a new emotional self-management program on stress, emotions, heart rate variability, DHEA and cortisol." *Integrative Physiological and Behavioral Science: The Official Journal of the Pavlovian Society* vol. 33,2 (1998): 151-70. doi:10.1007/BF02688660.

[59] Mahindru, Aditya et al. "Role of Physical Activity on Mental Health and Well-Being: A Review." *Cureus* vol. 15,1 e33475. 7 Jan. 2023, doi:10.7759/cureus.33475.

[60] Price, Colin. «ELF Electromagnetic Waves from Lightning: The Schumann Resonances.» *Atmosphere*, vol. 7, no. 9, 2016, p. 116. MDPI, https://doi.org/10.3390/atmos7090116.

[61] Chevalier, Gaétan et al. "Earthing: health implications of reconnecting the human body to the Earth›s surface electrons." *Journal of Environmental and Public Health* vol. 2012 (2012): 291541. doi:10.1155/2012/291541.

[62] Jung, Carl. *Dream Analysis: Notes on a Lecture Given in 1928-1930.* Edited by J. Campbell, Princeton University Press, 1989.

[63] Ulrich, R. S., Simons, R. F., Losito, B. D., Fiorito, E., Miles, M. A., and Zelson, M. (1991). "Stress recovery during exposure to natural and urban environments." *Journal of Environmental Psychology* 11(3), 201–230.

[64] Breus, Michael. *The Power of When: Discover Your Chronotype—and the Best Time to Eat Lunch, Ask for a Raise, Have Sex, Write a Novel, Take Your Meds, and More.* Little, Brown Spark, 2016.

[65] Brady, Tom. *The TB12 Method: How to Achieve a Lifetime of Sustained Peak Performance.* Simon & Schuster, 2017.

[66] Ross, Julia. *The Craving Cure: Identify Your Craving Type to Activate Your Natural Appetite Control.* Flatiron Books, 2017.

[67] Scheller, Brooke. How to Eat to Change *How You Drink: Heal Your Gut, Mend Your Mind, and Improve Nutrition to Change Your Relationship with Alcohol.* Balance, 2023.

Upgrade Your Epigenetics

[68] Heijmans, Bastiaan T., et al. «Persistent Epigenetic Differences Associated with Prenatal Exposure to Famine in Humans.» *Proceedings of the National Academy of Sciences*, vol. 105, no. 44, 2008, pp. 17046-17049. National Academy of Sciences, doi:10.1073/pnas.0806560105.

[69] Alberts, Bruce et al. *Molecular Biology of the Cell.* 4th ed., Garland Science, 2002. "Chromosomal DNA and Its Packaging in the Chromatin Fiber." NCBI Bookshelf.

[70] Collins, Francis S, and Leslie Fink. "The Human Genome Project." *Alcohol Health and Research World* vol. 19,3 (1995): 190–195.

[71] Król, Magdalena, et al. «The Fetal Alcohol Spectrum Disorders—An Overview of Experimental Models, Therapeutic Strategies, and Future Research Directions.» *Children*, vol. 11, no. 5, 2024, doi:10.3390/children11050531.

[72] Di Emidio, Giovanna et al. "Pre-conceptional maternal exposure to cyclophosphamide results in modifications of DNA methylation in F1 and F2 mouse oocytes: evidence for transgenerational effects." *Epigenetics* vol. 14,11 (2019): 1057–1064. doi:10.1080/15592294.2019.1631111.

[73] Krishnan, Harish R et al. "The epigenetic landscape of alcoholism." *International Review of Neurobiology* vol. 115 (2014): 75–116. doi:10.1016/B978-0-12-801311-3.00003-2.

[74] Kerr, David C R et al. "Intergenerational influences on early alcohol use: independence from the problem behavior pathway." *Development and Psychopathology* vol. 24,3 (2012): 889–906. doi:10.1017/S0954579412000430.

[75] Bowers, Mallory E, and Rachel Yehuda. "Intergenerational Transmission of Stress in Humans." *Neuropsychopharmacology: Official Publication of the American College of Neuropsychopharmacology* vol. 41,1 (2016): 232–44. doi:10.1038/npp.2015.247.

[76] Ungerer, Michelle et al. "In utero alcohol exposure, epigenetic changes, and their consequences." *Alcohol Research: Current Reviews* vol. 35,1 (2013): 37–46.

[77] Nielsen, David A et al. "Epigenetics of drug abuse: predisposition or response." *Pharmacogenomics* vol. 13,10 (2012): 1149–60. doi:10.2217/pgs.12.94.

[78] Tiffon, Céline. "The Impact of Nutrition and Environmental Epigenetics on Human Health and Disease." *International Journal of Molecular Sciences* vol. 19,11 3425. 1 Nov. 2018, doi:10.3390/ijms19113425.

[79] Plaza-Diaz, Julio et al. "Impact of Physical Activity and Exercise on the Epigenome in Skeletal Muscle and Effects on Systemic Metabolism." *Biomedicines* vol. 10,1 126. 7 Jan. 2022, doi:10.3390/biomedicines10010126.

[80] Dee, Garrett et al. "Epigenetic Changes Associated with Different Types of Stressors and Suicide." *Cells* vol. 12,9 1258. 26 Apr. 2023, doi:10.3390/cells12091258.

[81] McCraty, Rollin, Mike Atkinson, Dana Tomasino, and Raymond Trevor Bradley. «The Coherent Heart: Heart–Brain Interactions, Psychophysiological Coherence, and the Emergence of System-Wide Order.» *HeartMath Research Center*, Institute of HeartMath, 2006.

[82] Zhang, Xiang, and Shuk-Mei Ho. "Epigenetics meets endocrinology." *Journal of Molecular Endocrinology* vol. 46,1 (2011): R11-32. doi:10.1677/jme-10-0053.

[83] Cunliffe, Vincent T. "The epigenetic impacts of social stress: how does social adversity become biologically embedded?." *Epigenomics* vol. 8,12 (2016): 1653–1669. doi:10.2217/epi-2016-0075.

[84] Gaine, Marie E et al. "Sleep Deprivation and the Epigenome." *Frontiers in Neural Circuits* vol. 12 14. 27 Feb. 2018, doi:10.3389/fncir.2018.00014.

[85] Woo, Vivienne, and Theresa Alenghat. "Epigenetic regulation by gut microbiota." *Gut Microbes* vol. 14,1 (2022): 2022407. doi:10.1080/19490976.2021.2022407.

[86] Larson, P. J., Zhou, W., Santiago, A., et al. "Associations of the Skin, Oral, and Gut Microbiome with Aging, Frailty, and Infection Risk Reservoirs in Older Adults." *Nature Aging*, vol. 2, 2022, pp. 941–955. Nature, doi:10.1038/s43587-022-00287-9.

How Eliminating Alcohol Grows Your Business and Your Wealth

[87] Ooms, Frédéric et al. "Entrepreneurial Neuroanatomy: Exploring Gray Matter Volume in Habitual Entrepreneurs." *Journal of Business Venturing Insights*, vol. 22, 2024.

[88] Frone, Michael R. «Alcohol Use and Workplace Absenteeism: Examining the Contributions of Impairment and Alcoholism.» *Journal of Applied Psychology*, vol. 91, no. 3, 2006, pp. 744-757.

[89] Curran, C., and Drummond, C. «Alcohol Consumption and Its Association with Job Turnover and Lower Career Achievement.» *Addiction*, vol. 101, no. 2, 2006, pp. 173-178.

[90] National Institute on Alcohol Abuse and Alcoholism. "What Are the U.S. Guidelines for Drinking?" *Rethinking Drinking*, U.S. Department of Health and Human Services.

[91] Topiwala, A., et al. "Moderate Alcohol Consumption as Risk Factor for Adverse Brain Outcomes and Cognitive Decline: Longitudinal Cohort Study." *BMJ*, vol. 357, 2017, p. j2353, doi:10.1136/bmj.j2353.

[92] American Addiction Centers. "How the Pandemic Has Impacted Relationships." *American Addiction Centers*, 8 Apr. 2021.

[93] "Alcohol and Aggression.» *Psychological Bulletin*, vol. 131, no. 4, 2005, pp. 490-512. American Psychological Association, doi:10.1037/0033-2909.131.4.490.

[94] "Alcohol›s Effects on Social Behavior.» *Journal of Studies on Alcohol and Drugs*, vol. 77, no. 4, 2016, pp. 625-634. doi:10.15288/jsad.2016.77.625.

[95] Homish, G.G., & Leonard, K.E. (2007). The drinking partnership and marital satisfaction: The longitudinal influence of discrepant drinking. *Journal of Consulting and Clinical Psychology*, 75(1), 43–51. https://doi.org/10.1037/0022-006X.75.1.43

[96] "How Families Can Help with Alcohol Addiction Recovery." *Family & Addiction Recovery*, December 20, 2019.

[97] Caetano, R et al. "Alcohol-related intimate partner violence among white, black, and Hispanic couples in the United States." *Alcohol Research & Health: The Journal of the National Institute on Alcohol Abuse and Alcoholism*, vol. 25,1 (2001): 58-65.

[98] Steele, Claude M., and Robert A. Josephs. «Alcohol Myopia: Its Prized and Dangerous Effects.» *American Psychologist*, vol. 45, no. 8, 1990, pp. 921-933. doi:10.1037/0003-066X.45.8.921.

[99] Mylett, Ed. "Blake Mycoskie: The Business of Changing Lives." *The Ed Mylett Show*.

[100] Suu Kyi, Aung San. *Freedom from Fear and Other Writings*. Penguin Books, 1991. Amazon.

[101] Munger, Charlie. "Charlie Munger›s Speech to the Harvard School, June 1986." *BizNews*, 13 June 1986.

[102] Ellison, T.J. *Software: An Intimate Portrait of Larry Ellison and Oracle*. Free Press, 2003. Amazon.

[103] Sweeney, Emily. "Why More People Are Saying No to Alcohol." CNN, 8 June 2019.

Cultivating Sustainable Joy

[104] Koob, George F., and Michael Le Moal. «Neurobiological Mechanisms for Opponent Motivational Processes in Addiction.» *Pharmacology Biochemistry and Behavior*, vol. 79, no. 3, 2004, pp. 513-529, doi:10.1016/j.pbb.2004.09.019.

[105] Dixon, Matthew L., and Kalina Christoff. «Cognitive Control, Emotional Value, and the Lateral Prefrontal Cortex.» *Frontiers in Psychology*, vol. 5, 2014, doi:10.3389/fpsyg.2014.00758.

[106] Gardner, Eliot L. "Addiction and brain reward and antireward pathways." *Advances in Psychosomatic Medicine* vol. 30 (2011): 22–60. doi:10.1159/000324065.

Your Step-by-Step Action Plan to Becoming Alcohol-Free

[107] Koob, George F., and Michel Le Moal. «Neurobiological Mechanisms for Opponent Motivational Processes in Addiction.» *Pharmacology Biochemistry and Behavior*, vol. 79, no. 3, 2004, pp. 513-529, doi:10.1016/j.pbb.2004.09.019.

Embracing the Uncomfortable Clarity of Your New Reality

[108] Wolf, Robb. *The Paleo Solution: The Original Human Diet*. Victory Belt Publishing, 2017.

[109] Manson, Mark. "I Quit Drinking Alcohol... But Did Not Expect This." YouTube, uploaded by Mark Manson, 30 Mar. 2023.

[110] Manson, Mark. *The Subtle Art of Not Giving a F*ck: A Counterintuitive Approach to Living a Good Life*. Kindle ed., HarperOne, 2016.

INDEX

Numbers

12-step programs, 31, 85, 206
4-7-8 Breathing Technique, 83

4S model, 165, 166, 168, 170

A

acceptance, 170
accountability, 59, 60, 172, 185, 186, 187, 188, 190, 205, 206
acetaldehyde, 20, 156
action plan, 177, 178, 188, 193
activation, 19, 28, 61
active listening, 200
adaptability, 41, 111, 112
adaptation, 28, 112
addiction, xv, 14, 31, 85, 98, 99, 114, 180, 191
adverse reactions, 30
advertisements, 10, 207
affirmations, 41, 42, 189, 190
after-work drinks, 151, 152
Aguiar, Steve, 35
alcohol abuse, 21, 99, 137
Alcohol Use Disorder (AUD), 5, 16
Alcoholics Anonymous (AA), 32
cultivating sustainable joy, 162
deepen your connections, 128, 136, 139

drinking in moderation, 28
epigenetics, 98, 99
how to tell if you have, xiii, xiv
key indicators, xv, xvi
alcohol-free alternatives, 147
Alcohol-Free Lifestyle. Sic Passim
alcoholic, 195
alcohol-free success stories, 64, 175
cultivating sustainable joy, 162
deepen your connections, 134, 149
growing your business and wealth, 116
how alcohol destroys your body, 17, 18, 20
how to tell if you have AUD, xiii, xiv
human and alcohol history, 7
key indicators of AUD, xv
why we drink, 4
Alcoholics Anonymous (AA), xxiii, 31, 32, 64, 204
alcoholism, 5, 85, 99, 162

alter ego, 60, 61

Alter Ego Effect, The, 60

amends, 204

American Addiction Centers, 32, 127

AMG method, 78, 79

amino acids, 85, 86

anger, 40, 138

antioxidants, 23

anxiety
    alcohol-free scenarios, 55
    alcohol-free success stories, 64,
        156
    AMG method, 78
    cultivating sustainable joy, 162,
        164, 165
    deepen your connections, 128,
        130, 140, 148
    epigenetics, 95, 98, 102

healing your body and brain, 72

how alcohol destroys your body,
    20, 21

how to refocus your mindset, 48,
    49

psychological factors behind
    alcohol consumption, 13

apps, 100, 187, 188

Ashwagandha, 88

assertiveness, 61

atherosclerosis, 18

Atomic Habits, 46, 181

attachment issues, 140

authenticity, 131

autonomic nervous system, 84

avoidance, 150, 165

awareness, 16, 79, 100, 168

B

Babson, Roger, 177

bacteria, 22, 104

balance, 20, 24, 85, 86, 101, 102, 104

bar, xix, 10, 50, 85, 120, 146, 147

beer, xvii, xx, xxi, 6, 7, 9, 10, 13, 16,
    18, 23, 47, 49, 51, 55, 56, 73, 150,
    212, 231

benefit-driven language, 62

benefits, xiv, 13, 59, 76, 90, 101, 151,
    152, 153, 157, 171, 184, 190, 191, 192

Big Alcohol, 8, 9

binge drinking, 136, 150

blood pressure, 18, 36, 80, 84

blood sugar, 19, 87, 88

blood-brain barrier, 72

blue-blocking glasses, 103

Blum, Dr. Kenneth, 85

body language, 61

body scan, 169

boredom, 48, 169, 198

boundaries, 57, 152, 153

Bourgeois, Ronnie, 91

Brady, Tom, 84

brain, xiii, xxiv, 69, 112
    alcohol-free scenarios, 59, 60
    Alcoholics Anonymous (AA), 32
    AMG method, 79
    Big Alcohol's influence, 10
    cultivating sustainable joy, 163,
        164, 165
    dissolving the illusion of pleasure,
        33
    dopamine, 15, 73
    embracing the uncomfortable
        clarity, 209
    epigenetics, 97, 103
    growing your business and
        wealth, 111

healing the effects of alcohol, 72, 74, 75, 76, 89

health, 71

Hollywood's glamorization of alcohol, 11

how alcohol destroys your body, 18, 20

how alcohol impacts cognitive performance, 74

how to refocus your mindset, 41, 42, 43, 44, 48

human and alcohol history, 8

nutritional strategies, 85, 86, 87, 88

psychological factors behind alcohol consumption, 13, 14

brain how to refocus your mindset, 48

brainwashing, 11

breathing exercises, 52, 84

Brown, Brené, xvii

Budweiser, xvii, xxi, 10

Buffett, Warren, xvii, 149

burnout, 150

business opportunities, 40

buzz, 53, 207

C

camaraderie, 7

cancer, xiv, 16, 19, 20, 23, 24, 53

cannabis, 25, 26

carcinogen, 20

cardiomyopathy, 18

cardiovascular diseases, 95, 98

cardiovascular system, 18

Cardone, Grant, 183

career, xi, xxiv
  action plan, 180
  embracing the uncomfortable clarity, 196, 197, 201, 202, 203
  epigenetics, 105
  growing your business and wealth, 113, 114, 120, 121, 122
  healing the body and brain, 73, 74, 76
  how alcohol destroys your body, 30
  human and alcohol history, 8
  why go alcohol-free, xxi, xxii

casual drinker, 5, 24

Centers for Disease Control and Prevention (CDC), xiv, 24

changes, xi, xii, xiii, xx, xxiv, 55, 58, 59, 60, 61, 62, 112, 130, 153
  action plan, 179, 180, 181, 186, 190, 191
  alcohol-free scenarios, 49, 53
  alcohol-free success stories, 37, 91, 107, 123, 124, 212
  Alcoholics Anonymous (AA), 31, 33
  AMG method, 79
  deepen your connections, 134, 135, 136, 137, 140, 142, 143, 144, 148
  dissolving the illusion of pleasure, 33
  dopamine's role, 15
  embracing the uncomfortable clarity, 198, 199, 202, 203, 204, 208, 210
  epigenetics, 94, 95, 96, 97, 98, 99, 100, 101, 103, 104, 105
  growing your business and wealth, 111, 112, 117
  healing the body and brain, 77, 78, 84, 90
  healing your body and brain, 72, 73

how alcohol destroys your body, 16, 20, 24

how to refocus your mindset, 39, 41, 42, 46

how to tell if you have AUDs, xiii

key indicators of AUD, xviii

nutritional strategies, 87, 89

sharing your decision to stop, 132, 133, 143

why go alcohol-free, xxiii

why we drink, 5

check-ins, 82, 187, 201

Chromium Picolinate, 88

chronic alcohol abusers, 17

chronic drinking, 75

circadian rhythm, xx

cirrhosis, 17

clarity, xix, xxv
    4S model, 165
    action plan, 189
    alcohol-free success stories, 38, 175, 194
    cultivating sustainable joy, 163, 166, 168, 171, 172, 173
    deepen your connections, 148, 149, 151
    dissolving the illusion of pleasure, 34
    embracing the uncomfortable, 195, 196, 197
    embracing uncomfortable, 198, 199, 200, 201, 202, 210
    growing your business and wealth, 111, 113, 116, 118, 122
    healing the body and brain, 76

Clear, James, 46, 181

Clooney, George, 58

coaching, xxii, 5, 16, 91, 111, 129, 185, 186, 188, 208

cocaine, 25, 26, 27

cocktails, xvii, xx, 110

cognitive abilities, 111

cognitive decline, 16, 20, 71, 95, 102

cognitive function, 101, 103, 128

collagen, 23

comfort zone, xxii, 80

commitment, xx, 92
    action plan, 178, 180, 182, 183, 186, 187, 188, 190, 192
    alcohol-free success stories, 123
    cultivating sustainable joy, 171, 173
    deepen your connections, 130, 143
    embracing the uncomfortable clarity, 205, 206
    how to refocus your mindset, 45

community, xii, xiii, xxv
    action plan, 186, 188, 189, 190
    alcohol-free scenarios, 54, 59
    alcohol-free success stories, 123, 157
    Alcoholics Anonymous (AA), 31, 32
    deepen your connections, 144, 146
    epigenetics, 103
    healing the body and brain, 81
    how alcohol destroys your body, 21, 27
    how to tell if you have AUD, xiii
    why go alcohol-free, xxiii

compassion, 167, 168, 169, 170, 199, 205, 210

competitive advantage, 57, 70

confidence, 58, 61, 111, 131, 137, 191, 194, 203, 206, 208

conflicts, 128, 129, 131, 136, 139

confusion, 40, 137, 140, 141

connections, 41, 42, 82, 103, 107, 125, 127, 130, 146, 153, 165, 179, 188, 190

consequences, xxii, 16, 24, 49, 50, 71, 95, 98, 128, 129

conversation starters, 131, 139, 140, 146, 150

conversations, xx, 40, 56, 127, 133, 135, 140, 144, 183, 190, 199, 200

Cooper, Bradley, xviii

coordination, 72

coping mechanisms, 34, 136, 139, 140, 165, 169

cortisol, 101

counseling, 30, 131, 201

COVID-19, 24

coworkers, 121, 152, 153, 171

crack, 25, 26, 27, 28, 42

Craving Cure, The, 85

cravings
  4S model, 165, 168, 169, 170
  AMG method, 78
  cultivating sustainable joy, 166, 167
  dopamine's role, 15
  healing the body and brain, 78, 84
  how alcohol destroys your body, 16
  how to refocus your mindset, 44
  nutritional strategies, 85, 86, 87, 88
  psychological factors behind alcohol consumption, 13

creative outlets, 81

crystal meth, 25, 26

cues, 46, 47, 48, 49, 50, 51, 53, 58, 128, 129, 181

cultural conditioning, xvii

culture, xiii, 8, 28, 53, 127, 128, 150, 153, 207, 208

Cunningham, Bill, 175

curiosity, 151

cutting back, 25, 114, 134, 188

D

danger, xi, 18, 30

dating, xx, 130

decision-making, 15, 20, 72, 76, 111, 112, 122

dehydration, 85

delayed gratification, 163, 164

delayed reaction times, 73

Dell, Michael, xvii

dementia, 20, 71

dependence, xv, 21, 23, 27, 30, 87

depression, 20, 21, 40, 72, 73, 86, 98, 118, 120, 162, 175

deprivation, 62

detoxification, 17, 88

developmental issues, 24

diabetes, 19, 95, 98

Diet Cure, The, 85

diets, 7, 97

digestion, 19

disabilities, 24, 97

discomfort, 13, 164, 167, 168, 169, 183, 211

disulfiram (Antabuse), 30

diuretic, 85

DLPA (DL-Phenylalanine), 86

DNA, 20, 23, 89, 94, 95, 96, 97, 99, 100

Dodes, Dr. Lance, 31

dopamine, 14, 15, 73, 86, 163, 164, 230

drugs, 15, 25, 26, 27, 28, 30, 94, 128

drunkenness, 3, 109

Dry January, xiii, 209

DSM, xv, xvi, 21

Duhigg, Charles, 14, 47, 186

Dutch Hunger Winter, 94

dysregulation, 98, 140

E

early childhood development, 97

electrolytes, 85

Ellison, Larry, xvii, 150

emotional availability, 137, 140

emotional stability, 101

emotions, 91, 183
  alcohol-free success stories, 91
  cultivating sustainable joy, 162, 164, 165, 168, 169, 173
  deepen your connections, 126, 139, 141
  embracing the uncomfortable clarity, 199, 200, 205, 207, 210
  healing the body and brain, 78, 81
  healing your body and brain, 72
  Hollywood's glamorization of alcohol, 11
  how to tell if you have AUD, xiii
  why go alcohol-free, xxii

empathy, 82, 83, 128, 199, 200

Empire Strikes Back, 45

endorphins, 53, 78, 79, 86

energy, xx, xxi
  action plan, 179, 180, 182, 183, 186, 189, 190
  alcohol-free scenarios, 55, 60
  alcohol-free success stories, 123, 124
  AMG method, 79
  cultivating sustainable joy, 167, 172, 173
  deepen your connections, 126, 137, 152
  embracing the uncomfortable clarity, 197, 199, 202
  epigenetics, 100
  growing your business and wealth, 110, 113, 114, 115, 116, 118, 120, 121, 122
  healing the body and brain, 75, 76, 77, 78, 82, 90
  healing your body and brain, 70, 71
  how alcohol destroys your body, 24
  how to refocus your mindset, 39
  key indicators of AUD, xviii
  nutritional strategies, 86, 87, 88
  routines, 52
  why go alcohol-free, xxi, xxiii
  why we drink, 5

enjoyment, 5, 164, 203

entrepreneurs, xxiv, 42, 50, 56, 70, 110, 111, 112, 113, 126, 149

environment
  how to refocus your mindset, 48

Environment
  action plan, 181, 183, 188, 189
  alcohol-free scenarios, 49, 50
  Alcoholics Anonymous (AA), 32
  deepen your connections, 138
  epigenetics, 97, 99, 102, 104, 105
  growing your business and wealth, 112
  how alcohol destroys your body, 30

environmental factors, 94, 95, 104

epigenetics, 89, 93–109

erectile dysfunction (ED), 23, 86, 130, 205

escape, 14, 48, 51, 73, 139, 147, 204

estrogen, 101, 102

ethanol, 20

euphoria, 79

events, xxii, 10, 14, 42, 47, 53, 57, 116, 127, 134, 146, 150, 189, 190, 207

executives, xxiv, 5, 50, 56, 75

exercise, xx, 43, 78, 79, 100, 102, 170, 171, 180, 189, 191, 205

Eyal, 11

F

Facebook, 11, 150, 187

family, xii, xx, 53, 55, 59, 82, 92, 127
  action plan, 180, 185, 187, 189
  alcohol-free success stories, 91, 123, 156, 157
  Big Alcohol's influence, 10
  cultivating sustainable joy, 171
  deepen your connections, 127, 136, 138, 143
  embracing the uncomfortable clarity, 197, 198, 208
  epigenetics, 99, 100, 102, 105, 106
  growing your business and wealth, 121
  healing the body and brain, 82
  how alcohol destroys your body, 16, 27
  how to refocus your mindset, 40
  how to tell if you have AUD, xiv
  human and alcohol history, 7
  key indicators of AUD, xvi, xviii
  taking your power back, 63
  why go alcohol-free, xxii, xxiii
  why we drink, 5

fatigue, 50, 75, 91

fatty liver, 17

fear, xix, xxii, 10, 40, 41, 112, 137, 138, 150, 162, 197

Ferrazzi, Keith, 59, 145

fertility, 24

fetal alcohol syndrome, 24

fibrosis, 17

fight or flight, 64

financial security, 203

fitness, 52, 100, 102, 126, 173, 190, 194, 209

Fitzgerald, F. Scott, 125

FMRI neuroimaging scans, 42

Foundation for Alcohol Research, 9

freedom, xiii, 64, 65, 145, 179, 194, 207

Freedom from Fear, 145

fulfillment, xviii, 5, 105, 154, 163, 164, 172, 173, 174, 202, 203, 210, 211

fun, xx, xxv, 7, 61
  alcohol-free scenarios, 54, 55, 56, 57, 60
  alcohol-free success stories, 107
  Big Alcohol's influence, 10
  cultivating sustainable joy, 164, 166, 174
  deepen your connections, 128, 132, 134, 135, 140, 141, 142, 146, 147, 148, 152
  embracing the uncomfortable clarity, 207
  healing the body and brain, 81
  how alcohol destroys your body, 23
  how to refocus your mindset, 42, 43
  human and alcohol history, 8
  nutritional strategies, 88

G

GABA, 73, 74, 86, 88

Gaines, Jessica, 107

genes, 94, 95, 96, 98, 101, 103, 104

Genius Foods, 71

Genius Life and Genius Kitchen, 71

glutamate, 74

glutamine, 86, 88

glutathione, 88

goals, 151, 201

action plan, 183, 187, 188, 190, 191, 192
alcohol-free scenarios, 59
alcohol-free success stories, 91
cultivating sustainable joy, 163, 174
deepen your connections, 135, 151
embracing the uncomfortable clarity, 200, 201
growing your business and wealth, 112, 121, 122
healing the body and brain, 82
Golden Globes, 70

gout, 36
gratitude, 77, 78, 79, 101, 171
Gray, Tim, 29
Greenfield, Ben, 28
grief, 175, 199
grounding, 78, 80
Grundhofer, Karen, 64
Grüvi, 54
guilt, 205
gut, 22, 104
Guthrie, Thomas, 69

H

habits, xii, 34, 53, 58, 189
action plan, 180, 181, 191, 192
cultivating sustainable joy, 171, 173
deepen your connections, 134, 146
embracing the uncomfortable clarity, 209
epigenetics, 99, 100
growing your business and wealth, 110, 112, 113, 114, 115, 117, 121
healing your body and brain, 70, 71
how alcohol destroys your body, 30
how to refocus your mindset, 45, 46, 47, 49
key indicators of AUD, xv, xvii
psychological factors behind alcohol consumption, 14
why go alcohol-free, xxiii
hangover, xviii, xix, 78
Hansen, Christina, 204
happiness, xiii, xvii, xviii, xxiv, 11, 60, 62, 77, 86, 118, 120, 163, 164, 171
happy hours, 150
Harbinger, Jordan, 196
healing, 32, 64, 69, 78, 143, 144, 163, 164, 165, 183, 204, 205

health, xi, xx, xxiv, 70
action plan, 182, 189, 191
alcohol-free scenarios, 50, 59
alcohol-free success stories, 91, 123, 156, 157, 175
Big Alcohol's influence, 9
cultivating sustainable joy, 171
deepen your connections, 127, 131, 151, 153
dopamine's role, 15, 16
embracing the uncomfortable clarity, 196, 200, 208
epigenetics, 94, 95, 97, 98, 99, 102, 104, 106
growing your business and wealth, 111, 120
healing the body and brain, 77, 90
healing your body and brain, 70, 71
how alcohol destroys your body, 16, 17, 20, 22, 23, 28, 29
how to tell if you have AUD, xiv
key indicators of AUD, xvi, xviii
nutritional strategies, 87, 88
psychological factors behind alcohol consumption, 13
taking your power back, 62
why go alcohol-free, xxiii

heart, xvi, 8, 9, 16, 18, 59, 72, 77, 84, 101, 102, 157, 162, 167, 170, 199

heartburn, 22

heavy drinking, 17, 22, 99, 182

Hebb, Dr. Donald, 43, 48

Helmstetter, Shad, 41

helplessness, 40

hepatitis, 17

herbal teas, 50, 189

Herman, Todd, 60

heroin, 25, 26, 27, 28

high performers, xii, xviii, 5, 70, 111, 149

hippocampus, 71, 72

hobbies, 174, 189, 191

Holiday, Ryan, 165

Hollywood, xviii, 10, 110

home detox, 50

hormesis, 28, 29

hormones, 18, 72, 84, 101, 102

hospitality, 7

How to Eat to Change How You Drink, 87

Huffington, Arianna, xvii, 149

hydration, 100

hypertension, 18

hypothalamus, 72

I

identity, xxii, 60, 61, 194, 202

immune function, 22, 83, 103

immune system, 16, 22, 59, 88, 104, 120

impaired motor skills, 73

impulse control, 15, 138

indoctrination, 55

inflammation, 17

inhibitions, 128, 131, 138

insecurity, 162

insomnia, 83, 120

inspiration, xiii, 73, 75

insulin, 19, 101, 102

insulin resistance, 19

integrity, 185, 199, 206

intention, xxi, 43, 44, 45, 54, 56, 57, 143, 148, 189

International Agency for Research on Cancer (IARC), 19

International Diabetes Federation, 19

introspection, 48

irritability, 86, 127, 128, 138

isolation, 59, 102, 107

J

Johnson, Dwayne, 58

journaling, 52, 81, 168, 188, 200

joy, xxv
  4S model, 165, 170
  alcohol-free success stories, 64
  cultivating, 161, 162, 164, 166, 171, 174
  deepen your connections, 146, 154
  embracing the uncomfortable clarity, 207, 210
  epigenetics, 101
  healing the body and brain, 81

judgment, 76, 135, 151, 167, 168, 170, 202

Jung, Carl, 79, 161

K

Kan, Justin, 150

Keltner, John, 212

Kombucha, 54, 182, 232, 233

Kyi, Aung San Suu, 145

L

language patterns, 41, 43

leaders, xvii, 9, 111, 149

leaky gut syndrome, 22

Lijphart, Anna, 194

liver, 16, 17, 19, 22, 59, 85, 87

loneliness, 102, 107, 169

longevity, xiii, 29

Lopez, Jennifer, xviii, xxi, 110

loving-kindness phrases, 170

L-Theanine, 88

Lugavere, Max, 71

M

Mad Men, 10, 11

magnesium, 22, 85, 88

Manson, Mark, 198, 204

marketing, 10, 12, 75, 110

McCraty, Rollin, 77

meaningful connections, 126, 155

Medication-Assisted Treatment (MAT), 30

medications, 30, 36, 86, 156

medicine, xiii, 31, 36, 114, 162

mediocrity, xix, 40

meditation, 52, 53, 101, 165, 166, 171, 191

Melcher, Evan, 156

memory, xvi, 16, 20, 72, 73, 83

menstrual cycles, 24

mental health, 20, 79, 95, 98, 101, 114

metabolic disorders, 95

Methylated B Vitamin Complex, 88

migraines, xix

Mind, body and spirit, 24

mindfulness, 44, 52, 101, 163, 165, 166, 173

mindset, 33, 39, 46, 49, 62, 63, 112, 145, 173, 189, 190

mistakes, 59

misuse, xiii, 25, 128

mitochondrial function, 28, 29

mocktails, 46, 50, 189

  Apple-Cucumber-Celery Smoothie, 233

  Cherry Pomegranate Seltzer, 234

  Classic Cider, 232

  Classic Sparkling Lemon Water, 225

  Cleansing Ginger-Cucumber-Mint Drink, 228

  Cranberry Berry Smash, 236

  Cranberry Fizz, 230

  Cranberry Sunrise Sparkler, 234

  Flavored Soda Water, 232, 233

  Ginger Ale and Lemon, 234

  Ginger Spice Fizz, 224

  Hot Honey Tea, 230

  Lime-Cucumber-Mint Water, 235

  Perrier Cranberry, 226

  Sparkling Cranberry-Lime Water, 228

  Sparkling Rosé Mocktail, 232

  Specialty Infused Sparkling Water, 231

  Virgin Mojito, 226, 228

moderate drinking, xiv, 10, 119
money, xix, xxv, 9, 10, 50, 52, 70, 111, 114, 115, 117, 120, 179, 185, 207
mood, 36, 52, 56, 72, 78, 80, 85, 86, 88, 118, 128, 129, 137, 190
Mood Cure, The, 85
mortality, 19, 24, 27

motivation, xiii, xviii, xxi, 73, 115, 139, 151, 180, 188, 190
movement, 78, 79, 100
movies, 4, 10, 182
Munger, Charlie, 149
Murthy, Dr. Vivek, xiv
Muscara, Cory, 165, 166, 167
Mycoskie, Blake, xvii, 130

N

NAC (N-Acetyl Cysteine), 88
naltrexone, 30
National Institute on Alcohol Abuse and Alcoholism, 9
National Institutes of Health, 84
nature, 78, 79, 80, 97, 123, 183, 191
nausea, xvi
negative effects, 99, 194
negative emotions, 14, 48, 165
neural connections, 41
neurological problems, 16
neurons, 41, 43, 71
neuropathy, 20, 175
neuroplasticity, 40, 41
neuroscience, xiii, 32, 33, 172

neurotransmitters, 72, 73
Never Eat Alone, 59, 145
nicotine, 25, 26, 166
Nielsen data, xvii
night sweats, xix
Non-Alcoholic Beer & Sparkling Water, 230
nonalcoholic drinks, 57
normalized behavior, 47
numbing, 30, 164, 171, 196, 199
nutrient absorption, 22
nutrients, 22, 85, 87, 88
nutrition, 85, 87, 100, 171, 173
nutritional therapy, 85
Nutt, Dr. David, 27

O

Obstacle Is the Way, The, 40, 165
obstacles, 112, 113
Omega-3, 87, 88

online communities, 187
Owens, Terrell, 70

P

painkiller, 165
Paleo Solution, The, 179
pancreas, 16, 19
pancreatitis, 19
parties, 7, 70, 127

peer pressure, 7
perception, 7, 8, 10, 34, 40, 101
perfection, 81, 144, 192
performance, xxiv, 61, 124
    alcohol-free scenarios, 60

cultivating sustainable joy, 166

deepen your connections, 149

growing your business and wealth, 111, 112, 113, 115

healing the body and brain, 74, 75, 89

healing the effects of alcohol, 89

healing your body and brain, 70

how alcohol destroys your body, 23

key indicators of AUD, xviii

psychological factors behind alcohol consumption, 13

personal development, xxiv, 71, 151, 171, 191

personal growth, 148, 191, 196

physical abnormalities, 97

physical activity, 78

pleasure, xvi, 13, 14, 30, 33, 48, 73, 163, 164, 173

poison, xvii, 4, 16, 29, 55, 56, 58, 71, 89, 162, 175, 208

Portman, Natalie, xviii

positive reinforcement, 14, 48

positive thinking, 42

Power of Habit, The, 14, 186

Power of When, The, 83

prayer, 52, 101, 124

prefrontal cortex, 15

pregnancy, 24, 97

premature ejaculation, 23

problem-solving, 72

procrastination, 75

productivity, xx, 91, 110, 111, 120, 122, 150

professional guidance, 191

professional situations, 57

professionals, xxiv, 5, 13, 17, 33, 50, 74, 111, 162, 184, 186, 203

progress, xxv, 4, 17, 71, 170, 188, 190, 192

progressive muscle relaxation, 169

Project 90, xi

action plan, 184, 186, 188

alcohol-free success stories, 107, 194, 212

deepen your connections, 127, 131, 136

embracing the uncomfortable clarity, 204, 208

growing your business and wealth, 113

healing your body and brain, 73

how alcohol destroys your body, 16, 18, 21

why go alcohol-free, xxii

protein, 87, 96, 233

psoriasis, 23

psychological diseases, xv

psychological factors, 33, 185

PTSD, 95, 98

purpose, 57, 61, 91, 123, 173, 180, 183

Q

quality of life, 117, 120, 172, 207

quick start, 178, 188

R

reasons for quitting, 191

recipes, 100, 134, 223

recovery, 32, 90, 99, 103

Reddit, 187

regrets, 136, 147, 204, 205

rehabilitation programs, 30

relationships, xi, xx, xxv, 34, 92
    action plan, 179, 189
    alcohol-free scenarios, 59
    alcohol-free success stories, 91
    deepen your connections, 127, 128, 131, 136, 144, 145, 146, 148, 149, 153, 155
    dopamine's role, 16
    embracing the uncomfortable clarity, 196, 197, 198, 199, 203, 205, 206, 211
    growing your business and wealth, 110, 120
    healing the body and brain, 82
    how alcohol destroys your body, 27
    taking your power back, 62
    why go alcohol-free, xxii, xxiii
    why we drink, 5
relaxation, 14, 48, 88, 107, 169
relief, 11, 13, 21, 37, 48, 49, 77, 81, 86, 103, 199
Renaud, Serge, 8
reproductive issues, 95
reprogramming, 42, 209
research
    action plan, 179
    Big Alcohol's influence, 9
deepen your connections, 128
drinking in moderation, 25
embracing the uncomfortable clarity, 203
epigenetics, 97, 99, 101
growing your business and wealth, 111, 114, 120
Hollywood's glamorization of alcohol, 11
how alcohol destroys your body, 17, 18, 19, 28, 29
how to refocus your mindset, 42
how to tell if you have AUD, xiv
nutritional strategies, 85
why go alcohol-free, xxiii
resilience, 28, 64, 101, 210
responsibility, 99, 102, 204, 205, 206
restlessness, xvi
reticular activating system (RAS), 43
reward, 14, 46, 48, 49, 53, 163, 190
ripple effect, 28, 89, 153, 171, 173
rituals, 6, 61, 77, 134
Robbins, Tony, xvii, 171
rock bottom, xv, xix, xxiii, 204
rosacea, 23
routine, 14, 24, 46, 48, 51, 52, 77, 102, 103, 140, 189

S

sadness, 35, 48, 139
Safer, Morley, 8
safety, 138
satisfaction, 128, 153, 163, 164, 203, 207
Sawni, Niki and Anika, 54
Scheller, Dr. Brooke, 87
schizophrenia, 95
Schumann resonance, 78
science, xiii, xxiii, 10, 14, 31, 46, 62, 89, 94, 111
sedentary behavior, 42
self-awareness, 48, 115, 180
self-care, 191
self-control, 163
self-discipline, xix, xx
self-esteem, 194, 208
self-loathing, 194
self-talk, 41, 42, 44, 46, 169, 189

Seneca, 3

Sex, xvi, 10, 15, 164, 198, 207

sexual and reproductive health, 23

shakiness, xvi

Shawcross, Dr. Debbie, 17

Shoes, Toms, xvii, 130

Simpsons, The, 49

skills, 53, 72, 80, 89, 118, 128, 131, 203

skin, xix, 22, 23, 80, 104, 124

sleep, xx, xxii, 13, 43, 72, 77, 83, 88, 102, 103, 111, 114, 124, 137, 157, 190, 212

slurred speech, 73

Smiling Assassins, 54

Smith, Dr. Bob, 31

Smith, Will, 178, 185

sober living, 187, 188

Sober October, xiii, 209

Sober Truth, The, 31

sobriety, 64, 118

social anxiety, 126, 148

Social Cognitive and Affective Neuroscience, 42

social standing, 7

socializing, 42, 128, 146, 155, 190

society, 4, 63, 123, 164, 183

Socrates, 39

soda, xix, 18, 46, 54, 57, 58, 184, 224, 226, 234, 235, 236

softening, 167, 169

sperm, 97

stability, 137, 138

stigma, xxiii, 33

stimulation, 14, 164

stimuli, 42, 181

Stockwell, Tim, 9

stomach ulcers, 22

Stop Missing Your Life, 165

strategies, 33, 76, 83, 87, 183, 191

stress, xii, 50
    action plan, 189
    alcohol-free scenarios, 50, 52, 59
    alcohol-free success stories, 37
    cultivating sustainable joy, 162, 164, 169
    deepen your connections, 126, 128, 136, 139
    dissolving the illusion of pleasure, 34
    embracing the uncomfortable clarity, 204
    epigenetics, 94, 97, 98, 101, 103
    growing your business and wealth, 112, 115
    healing the body and brain, 75, 77, 78, 80, 81, 82, 84
    how alcohol destroys your body, 19, 28, 29
    how to refocus your mindset, 48, 49
    nutritional strategies, 86, 88, 89

Stress
    Hollywood's glamorization of alcohol, 12
    how alcohol destroys your body, 18
    how to tell if you have AUD, xiii
    psychological factors behind alcohol consumption, 12, 13, 14

stroke, 18

studies. See research, 9, 11, 18, 21, 22, 23, 25, 27, 31, 42, 55, 58, 72, 80, 84, 102, 119, 128, 165

substance abuse, 31

substance use, 98, 139

success stories, 35, 36, 37, 38, 64, 65, 91, 92, 107, 123, 124, 156, 157, 175, 194, 212, 213

suffering, xi, 94

supplements, 85, 86, 88

suppor
  nutritional strategies, 86
support, xiii, xxv, 102, 188
  action plan, 182, 185, 186, 187, 188,
    189, 190, 191, 193
  alcohol-free scenarios, 59
  alcohol-free success stories, 35,
    64
  Alcoholics Anonymous (AA), 31
  deepen your connections, 132, 137,
    141, 142, 143, 145, 150
  embracing the uncomfortable
    clarity, 200, 206
  epigenetics, 99, 104

  growing your business and
    wealth, 119
  healing the body and brain, 77, 82,
    83, 90
  how alcohol destroys your body,
    30
  nutritional strategies, 87
Swanwick Sleep, 103, 111
Swanwick, Edward and Tristan, xxv,
  103, 111
Symonds, Matthew, 150
symptoms, xv, xvi, 90, 150, 165
synaptic plasticity, 74

T

TB12 Method, The, 84
teasing, 147
television, 4, 10, 182
temptation, 8, 49
testosterone, 101, 102
therapy, 30
thought patterns, 30, 41, 50, 51
tolerance, 15, 163
tools, xii, 62, 64, 154, 186, 188
top performers, 8, 19, 29, 30, 40, 42,
  50, 56
toxins, 22, 85, 114, 162, 171
training, 36, 203

transformation, xv, xvii, xxiii, 49, 61,
  107, 126, 166, 172, 196
transgressions, 204
transition, 135, 178, 203
trauma, xxiii, 64, 98, 204
treatment, 31, 32, 99
triggers, 11, 34, 47, 50, 51, 77, 169, 181,
  189
trust, 82, 129, 131, 137, 138, 139, 142,
  144, 147, 184, 187, 202, 210
tryptophan, 86
Turner, Thomas, 9
tyrosine, 86

U

unpredictability, 138

urges, 30

V

vascular damage, 23
vitality, 107, 182
vitamin deficiencies, 87
vitamins, 23, 87
volunteer organizations, 82

vulnerability, 82, 91, 205

W

water, xix, xx
  action plan, 182, 189
  alcohol-free scenarios, 54, 58
  deepen your connections, 134, 151
  healing the body and brain, 84, 85
  how alcohol destroys your body, 29
  how to refocus your mindset, 46
  human and alcohol history, 7
Watts, Alan, 162
wealth, xxiii, 62, 91, 105, 109
weight, xviii, 13, 37, 75, 84, 91, 112, 124, 194, 206, 213
What to Say When You Talk to Yourself, 41
whiskey, 10, 23, 49, 212
why we drink, 3, 33
Williams, Pharrell, xviii
Williams, Robin, 195
willpower, 185
Wilson, Bill, 31
Wilt, Steve, 123

wine, xii, xx, 16, 127
  alcohol-free scenarios, 50
  alcohol-free success stories, 157
  Big Alcohol's influence, 8, 9, 10
  deepen your connections, 130
  dopamine's role, 16
  growing your business and wealth, 110, 116, 119, 120
  healing the body and brain, 75
  how alcohol destroys your body, 18, 21, 23
  how to refocus your mindset, 47, 48, 49
  human and alcohol history, 7
  key indicators of AUD, xvii
  psychological factors behind alcohol consumption, 13
Wisdom of Insecurity, The, 162
withdrawal symptoms, xvi, xix, 13, 30
Wolf, Robb, 179
work quality, 75
wrinkles, 22

Y

yoga, 52, 146, 191

YouTube, 53, 198